SOCIAL WORK SERVICES AND PATIENT DECISION MAKING

Social Work Services and Patient Decision Making

PATRICIA HANSEN
Family and Children's Services
Western Australia

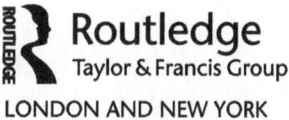
Routledge
Taylor & Francis Group

LONDON AND NEW YORK

First published 1998 by Ashgate Publishing

Reissued 2018 by Routledge
2 Park Square, Milton Park, Abingdon, Oxon, OX14 4RN
711 Third Avenue, New York, NY 10017, USA

Routledge is an imprint of the Taylor & Francis Group, an informa business

Notice:
Product or corporate names may be trademarks or registered trademarks, and are used only for identification and explanation without intent to infringe.

Publisher's Note
The publisher has gone to great lengths to ensure the quality of this reprint but points out that some imperfections in the original copies may be apparent.

Disclaimer
The publisher has made every effort to trace copyright holders and welcomes correspondence from those they have been unable to contact.

A Library of Congress record exists under LC control number: 97077389

ISBN 13: 978-1-138-34346-7 (hbk)
ISBN 13: 978-1-138-34350-4 (pbk)
ISBN 13: 978-0-429-43911-7 (ebk)

Contents

Figures and tables

Foreword

Patients and their families have always been faced with the task of making decisions about treatment, discharge plans, and other medical concerns during hospital stays. What makes the task so much more difficult in today's medical environment is the complexity and rapidly changing nature of health care systems. These changes have resulted in decisions being made under great time constraints and emotional duress. In light of the shorter lengths of stay in the hospital and a move toward a capitated reimbursement system, social workers must be knowledgeable about effective interventions for a clientele with an array of psychosocial needs. In addition, the downsizing of social work departments forces administrators to calculate carefully the costing of services and how to allocate resources to increase worker productivity.

Given these increasing pressures in medical settings, Dr Hansen's work on decision making and cost analysis of social work services is particularly timely. Her critical analysis of decision making by patients and their families attends to many of the important factors that facilitate effective decisions. By directing interviewing patients and their families, her study enables us to listen to the voices of the recipients of our services and hear what facilitates or hinders their decision making.

Dr Hansen's application of activity based costing to social work services and the identification of cost drivers present a ground breaking analysis of social work services. Identifying cost drivers is a critical job for social work administrators as they attempt to allocate social work services within an environment of diminishing resources. Her study serves as an exemplar for future social work research in this area.

The findings of Dr Hansen's study present a valuable but sobering perspective on the effectiveness of social work practice in health care. In particular, she questions what can realistically be accomplished in such a brief period of time. She offers several sound suggestions that will help the profession to provide comprehensive and effective psychosocial services for our patients and families. For example, she makes a convincing argument for social workers to work with families of patients and not just the patients themselves. Also, she recommends moving some services back to the community. Needs do not end when patients are discharged. Indeed, sometimes it is when the patient returns home that the psychosocial issues and needs become most apparent. Dr Hansen's scholarly work on social work practice in health care is a very noteworthy contribution to our profession.

Karen Kayser, PhD
Associate Professor
Graduate School of Social Work
Boston College
May 1997

Social work practice in hospitals has changed markedly over recent years. The incorporation of business concepts into the health care service delivery and the funding of services has driven this change. Where before social work management was primarily concerned with balancing the budget at the end of the fiscal year there is now pressure on departments to demonstrate that expenditures result in positive outcomes for the organisation. Failure to do so may result in the weakening of social work services and reduced availability of social work services to patients and their families.

Given the pressures from the external environment, there is a need for more detailed and accurate costing information to effectively analyse costs incurred in service delivery in relation to the medical units within the hospital, and a need for an examination of costs in relation to output and outcomes. However, the elements of traditional cost accounting have been identified as too complex for human services (Vinter and Kish 1984) and management accounting systems have been described as not providing information that is usable by line managers in human services (Hairston 1985). The obstacles to analysing costs within the social work profession must be overcome if social work services in the health care system are to aid in the development of information systems that assist in the management of service delivery in the current environment.

Fortunately, Pat Hansen has made a major contribution to the hospital social work domain by introducing the use of activity based costing (ABC). Quite simply, the ABC approach is likely to be attractive to social workers because it focuses on tracing costs through activities. This results in a more accurate measurement of costs. For example, preparation and travel time are often significant costs that have been ignored, but through Hansen's work can now be traced to a particular social work service that has been provided.

In addition, Pat Hansen's work allows social workers to accurately identify cost drivers. For example, in this study, Hansen identified the following cost drivers for social work costs in one hospital in New England. They were length of stay, patients income level (inverse relationship), the existence of disagreement between the patient and family about the patient's discharge destination, and patient's concern about problems with employment or study. These characteristics of the patient and their circumstances are understable as cost drivers. It may be expected that people with lower incomes may experience more difficulties in meeting financial commitments when they are faced with serious illness, and they may also have fewer choices about the services they may access during the recovery period after discharge. In response to these difficulties, the social worker may be required to spend longer time in negotiation with potential service providers and with creditors. Similarly, the demands on social work time are inevitable when the family and patient do not agree about plans for the patient's future living arrangements, since the family is the primary source of post hospital care for most patients. Finally, difficulties with work or with educational institutions may require prolonged negotiation if the patient's capacity to resume their responsibilities is uncertain or markedly altered as a result of their illness or treatment.

As an accountant, I applaud Pat Hansen's work for trying to integrate such different disciplines as social work and accounting. If there can be a joint undertaking of cost analysis by social workers and accountants the results may be of benefit to all concerned. Social work practices and systems of service delivery may be altered by the knowledge obtained from such analyses. Certainly the information available to account for use of resources will be improved by professional costing exercises and this may benefit the organisation in funding or contract negotiations.

Pat Hansen has taken the crucial first step in helping social workers and accountants to engage in an effective dialogue where the interests of the ultimate client, the patient, will be honourably served.

Jeffrey R Cohen, PhD, CMA
Department Chair, Accounting
Carroll School of Management
Boston College
May 1997

Preface

This exploratory study examines i) the effect of the decision making environment on patient satisfaction and psychosocial outcomes, and ii) the impact of disagreements and type of patients' problems on social work time expenditure per patient.

A cross sectional survey approach was designed to compare the perceptions of 94 social work patients and 100 non social work patients about decision-making and outcomes. The structured interview schedule by which data were collected in telephone interviews included the validated decision-making scales developed by Coulton and colleagues (Coulton, Dunkle, Chow, Haug, and Vielhaber, 1988), and questions developed specifically for this study.

It was hypothesised that aspects which facilitate decision making -- certainty about outcomes, control over decisions, and family support -- would be associated with higher levels of patient satisfaction with decisions and better psychosocial outcomes. Factors which inhibit decision making -- hypervigilance, having restricted choices, being rushed, and having disagreements -- were expected to be inversely related to psychosocial outcomes. It was also hypothesised that the outcomes would be better for social work as compared with non social work patients. The final hypothesis was that disagreements and types and number of problems would increase the cost of the social work services provided.

Multiple regression analyses were used to test all hypotheses. In the process of data analysis it became clear that some of the assumptions about social work intervention and the pattern of difficulties experienced by patients were not accurate, at least for this group of patients. A major finding was that patients, particularly social work patients, experienced a higher level of difficulty in relation to psychosocial problems after discharge in comparison with their reports of problems experienced while in hospital. In addition it was found that only family support, and not the certainty about decision outcomes or control over decision making, showed a significant relationship with psychosocial outcomes.

While substantial numbers of patients reported having experienced disagreements with both hospital staff and with family members, most also indicated that these disagreements had not made their hospital stay or planning for the future difficult for them.

In relation to utilisation of social work resources the most important finding was that social workers are able to spend very little time with patients and families. The cost drivers identified in this study were length of stay in hospital, low income level and the existence of family disagreement about discharge destination.

The results of this study raise concerns about how social workers are allocated to work within the health system. For those patients who have more problems after discharge than while in the hospital, community based, rather than hospital based services, appear warranted. The attempt to identify cost drivers conducted in this study is a small beginning. Identification of cost drivers and development of outcome measurement in relation to social work services must be an ongoing concern for social work managers and policy makers to ensure continued funding for services.

Acknowledgements

Staff at Boston College – Karen Kayser, Woo Sik Chung and Jeffrey Cohen have given advice and support throughout the period of this study. Their contribution is much appreciated. I am grateful to the patients who gave their time and energy to answer the questions in this study with careful and thoughtful responses even when they were still recovering from their illness and the hospital treatment. I also owe a great deal to the social workers and all staff in the social work department of the hospital who put up with my intrusion into their busy working days. Both The Gerontologist journal and Professor Claudia Coulton agreed to allow publication of the decision making scales which were used in this study. It is Angie Hearn's word processing skills and the patient and experienced editorial staff at Ashgate who have put it all together to produce the book. Most of all I appreciate Frank Ainsworth's contribution. He has been so generous with his help on this project and with so many endeavours over the years.

Introduction

Changes to the health care system over the last decade have increased pressure on patients and their families as well as hospital staff. The changes in medical technology and service delivery systems have heightened the importance of quality of life and the social circumstances of patients who live independently in the community in spite of chronic illness and disability (Lawlor and Raube, 1995). Psychosocial outcomes have been recognised as of equal importance to the physical outcomes, especially as the time in the acute care hospital has become more brief, leaving the patient, family, and community based systems to provide home based care.

Patients are in the hospital for very short periods of time at a point in their lives when their physical problems place them under considerable stress. The inevitable crisis associated with hospital treatment is exacerbated by the time pressure and the need for decisions about treatment and post discharge arrangements to be made promptly. There is the potential for disagreements between the patient and their family members or among the patient, family and hospital personnel. Given this pressurised situation it is inevitable that disagreements occur and that decision making is less than optimal (Abramson, Donnelly, King, and Mailick, 1993).

As part of this scenario the hospital based social worker is often in a situation of assisting the patient and family to obtain information, and facilitating negotiations among patients, family, community agencies and hospital health care personnel so that decisions and implementation may proceed without delay. Social workers are likely to be engaged in complex negotiations and intervention aimed at clarifying roles and relationships between the patient and family and between patient, family and other health care providers (Abramson, 1990; Bergman et al.,1993). There is a need to understand the results of such intervention.

Some social work research has focused on the impact of discharge planning on patients and families (Clemens, 1995; Oktay, Steinwachs, Mamon, Bone, and Fahey, 1993; Proctor, Morrow-Howell, Albaz, and Weir, 1992) and the degree to which patients have maintained control in decision making (Coulton, Dunkle,

Chow, Haug, and Vielhaber, 1988; Coulton, Dunkle, Haug, Chow, and Vielhaber, 1989; Reinhardy, 1995). A few studies have refined the decision making focus with a concentration on disagreements in relation to discharge planning from the social workers' perspective (Abramson et al., 1993). However, there has been limited study of disagreements from the patient's perspective (Reinhardy, 1995) and no studies focused on the effectiveness of social work intervention to deal with disagreements.

There are indications that when disagreements or conflict occur there may be increased length of stay for the patient (Proctor, Morrow-Howell, and Lott, 1993). Increased length of stay has been identified as related to increased use of social work resources (Coulton, Keller, and Boone, 1985; Semke, Stowell, and Durgin, 1993) and increased costs to the hospital (Bray, Carter, Dobson, Watt, and Shortell, 1994). In addition, when disagreements occur there is the potential for negative impact on patient and family satisfaction (Proctor et al., 1992). In the end if the patient does not agree with hospital personnel there is increased likelihood of patient noncompliance with treatment regimes which has been associated with risk of re admission (Saffran and Phillips, 1989; Zook, Savickis, and Moore, 1980). All these potential effects confirm a need for the study of patient decision making processes where there is a focus on the impact of disagreements on the patient's well-being, the effectiveness of social work intervention in relation to disagreements, and the role decision making and disagreements play as cost drivers in relation to social work time expenditure and the patient's length of stay in the hospital.

Through a systematic examination of patient health care decision making processes and the effectiveness of social work intervention in relation to disagreements, social workers will obtain a better understanding of the nature and process of patient decision making and the impact of social work intervention when disagreements occur. This kind of information has the potential to modify social work interventions to improve outcomes for patients and increase patient satisfaction.

When outcomes are considered it is also important to consider the question of inputs. The pressures on the health care system to reduce expenditures have been passed on to all services within the health care system over more than a decade (Coulton, 1984; Rosko and Broyles, 1988; Scott, 1994). Within social work this push to economise has provoked a number of productivity studies and attempts to measure what drives utilisation of social work resources (Haber-Scharf, 1985: Keller, Domanski, Macks, Manley, and Winder, 1993; Ponto and Berg, 1992; Spano, Kiresuk, and Lund, 1977; Volland, 1980). One response to this pressure is to argue against the inequalities of the current health system and to lobby for increased services to the vulnerable and disadvantaged within the community (Keigher, 1993; Taira and Taira, 1991) but this cannot be the sole strategy. Like medicine, nursing, physical therapy and other health professions, social work must be involved in analysis of resource utilisation as well as outcomes. The

2

examination of cost drivers is needed to contribute to the understanding of elements of the patient situation that lead to increased use of social work resources.

The emphasis here is on decision making and disagreements from the patients' perspective with exploration of the impact of disagreements on the patient and on use of social work time and the costs of services. Therefore, the purposes of the study are:

- to examine aspects of decision making and the impact of the decision making environment on patients' satisfaction with decisions and the patients' psychosocial outcomes;

- to examine the impact of disagreements on patients and the effectiveness of social work intervention in relation to patient decision making and psychosocial outcomes, and

- to examine whether aspects of decision making or disagreements constitute major cost drivers in relation to use of social work resources in the hospital setting.

From this type of study there cannot be definitive results to guide practice or policy. The cross section survey design and the early stage of theoretical development of the major constructs means that the data produced will be of use in guiding further research effort and examining whether trends found in previous studies have been replicated for this sample. This study provides information about the patients' experience in the hospital and after discharge in today's managed care environment. The information about decision making and disagreement processes contributes to an understanding of the impact of rapid treatment and discharge from the patients' perspective. The second part of the study which is focused on examination of resource utilisation contains rarely available data on costing of social work services and utilisation of social work resources.

3

1 Literature review

Decision making

The study of decision making is a cross disciplinary enterprise with many different perspectives (Cuzzi, Holden, Grob, and Bazer, 1993; Plous, 1993). Given an assumption that humans are rational beings, ideal decision making may be defined as including consideration of all options and possible consequences before the decision is made (Hogarth, 1987; Homans, 1974). However, the limits on human rationality have long been recognised (March and Simon, 1958).

Studies of information processing examine the effect of memory processes, judgment processes and control processes in decision making and problem solving (Lachman, Mistler-Lachman, and Butterfield, 1979). Within cognitive-behavioral theory cognition is described as including cognitive structure, processes and content (Kendall, 1991). Cognitive structures may be defined as memory or templates and may function as a filter to new experiences and information. The cognitive procedures or processes consist of how the person perceives and interprets experiences, and the content is the information presented. The cognitive products which result from the processes are the meanings given to information, the attributions about the intent and the causal processes.

Individual goals and affect are incorporated into this cognitive model so that judgment, goals and affect are seen as influencing choices and conations (intention to act). There has been debate as to whether it is reasonable to define general personality traits as in a generalised locus of control (Rotter, 1966) but Ajzen (1991) proposes that it is more accurate to consider aggregations of specific behaviors over time. The argument is that through observations carried out in different situations and times the external influences cancel each other out and the aggregate behavior may be identified. From this point the Ajzen theory of planned behavior suggest that motivational factors (attitudes towards behavior), together with perceived behavioral control and perceived subjective norms, constitute intentions to act. It is considered that the intention to act influences the likelihood of the behavior occurring.

Against this background it is important to recognise that decision making may be at different levels and not all decisions are treated as worthy of comprehensive problem solving assessment of all aspects and options available. In fact, in many situations it is thought that individuals use *heuristics*, or decision rules, to simplify information and make choices among alternatives (Plous, 1993).

The presentation of human decision making from cognitive theories is consistent with the concept of *satisficing* in decision making as described by March and Simon (1958). People are described as capable of dealing with only part of the available information and thus rationality is bounded. This *bounded rationality* results in satisficing decisions which are *good enough* rather than optimal.

From another perspective decision making in organisations has been examined in instances where the results were defined as negative. Janis and Mann (1977) have examined the psychological processes of decision making with definition of stages of decision making particularly in relation to decisions which are difficult to make. In studying poor decision making their intention is to provide guidelines to improve the quality of decisions. One of the situations analysed by Janis included the circumstances in the National Aeronautics and Space Administration (NASA) at the time of the Challenger disaster. In that situation the interactional processes within the organisation promoted *groupthink* (Janis, 1982) rather than careful analysis of available information. The complexities of the situation were ignored in order to serve political goals and to comply with the expectations of senior management. As a result of their studies Janis and Mann (1992) differentiate between simple decision strategies and complex ones. Simple strategies are those which may be based on satisficing, affiliative (preserving harmony) or egocentric (serving one's own interests) motives. Complex decision systems may include use of computer modeling, expert systems or decision analysis (Turban, 1990).

Another contribution in this field is concerned with the impact time pressure and fear have on decision making (Svenson and Maule, 1993). Time pressure has been associated with increased sensitivity to negative information (Svenson and Edland, 1989) as well as resulting in reduced information exchange. The efficiency of negotiations and capacity to reach mutually satisfying conclusions has been found to be influenced by whether the context is conflictual or cooperative (Carnevale, O'Connor, and McCusker, 1993). In addition, time pressure may lead to faster agreement on decisions, earlier concession to others and lower demands being made (Carnevale et al., 1993). Fear and anxiety appears to interfere with consideration of options. Janis and Mann (1977) describe this anxiety as *hypervigilance* which they associate with avoidance of decision making or ineffective decision making.

Uncertainty in decision making has been defined as when 'the experience of not knowing which of a set of alternative states of nature has occurred or will occur' (Sniezek and Buckley, 1993, p. 88). It is the subjective perception of how much a

6

situation may be predicted and it is known that the individual may experience confidence or uncertainty both before and/or after the decision has been made. Although there is relatively little research in this area it has been found that increased time and effort in decision making may reduce subjective uncertainty (Bettman, Johnson, and Payne, 1990; Paese and Sniezek, 1991). There is also the proposition that uncertainty is not a completely negative influence on decision making since it may interrupt action and lead the individual to reconsider the options (Lipshitz, 1993). These contributions highlight the inter-relationships between time pressure and perception of the decision making environment in relation to certainty of outcomes and underline that these factors do influence both the process and outcomes of decisions.

Such examinations of decision making emphasise the complexities involved in reaching decisions even when conditions are conducive to careful analysis of options. In the situations facing patients and families in today's health care system there is often limited time, considerable stress and the uncertainties associated with illness.

Decision making, self-determination and disagreements in hospital settings

Patient and family decision making

'Clients' right to self-determination is a key social work value' (Abramson, 1988, p. 443). The importance of self-determination is ensconced in the Code of Ethics (National Association of Social Workers [NASW], 1990) and recognised in every sphere of social work activity. In hospital settings it has become an issue for discussion because of the constraints placed on patients and families in the decision making process, particularly in relation to discharge planning (Abramson, 1988; Coulton, et al., 1989; Proctor et al., 1993).

Abramson (1988) studied social workers' evaluation of the participation in discharge planning by 85 of their older patients. The social workers identified patient's condition as a factor in determining participation. Families were described as actively involved in discharge planning. In a number of cases social workers spent more time with family members than with patients in the decision making process, but this was dependent on whether the patient was competent to participate. However, a quarter of the patients who were competent to participate were identified as not controlling the discharge decision. This finding indicates a need for further exploration of patients decision making particularly from the patients' perspective. The importance of patient involvement in decision making is also confirmed in a study of patient and family satisfaction at the point of discharge (Proctor et al., 1992). Patient involvement in decision making was identified as a predictor of patient satisfaction. For families the important factor was that the patient or spouse was involved in the decision making. Where the patient was not able to make the decision and when family members other than spouse made the decisions there was less family satisfaction with the plan.

Coulton and colleagues (Coulton et al., 1988) developed a model of patient decision making using concepts from psychological studies of decision making (Foreman, 1964; Janis and Mann, 1977; Kelly et al., 1965; Klein and Hill, 1979; Wicklund, 1974). They confirmed a six factor model of patient's decision making based on a study of patients' perceptions after discharge. The six factors were hypervigilance, family support, restricted choice, certainty, control and rushed. The definitions are as follows:

- *Hypervigilance*: a generalised anxiety, panic or fear about the decision to be made

- *Family support*: family members support of the patient's decisions and planning

- *Restricted choice*: limitation on options available

- *Certainty*: knowledge of potential outcomes of decisions, the predictability of decisions

- *Control*: how much control patient has in decision making

- *Rushed*: being rushed or pressured into a decision

(Coulton et al., 1988).

The importance of family in decision making in either supporting the patient's decisions or in making decisions on behalf of patients was also confirmed in this study. In a subsequent study, Coulton and associates (Coulton et al., 1989) examined the six scales in relation to locus of control using regression analysis. The findings supported the notion that patient's expectation of control influences the degree of decision anxiety.

The development of these decision making scales was based on a strong conceptual foundation but there may be some criticisms of the study. The confirmatory factor analysis of the six latent variables was conducted using the same data as that used for the initial exploratory factor analysis which defined the six decision making factors. In addition the scales for certainty in decision making, being rushed, and being in control presented low reliabilities. While these scales have considerable potential value as instruments to measure patient decision making the limitations of the confirmatory analysis indicate that the analysis of the structure and reliability must be re-examined in future studies.

Disagreements: patient, family and hospital staff

The pressured acute hospital arena seems designed to produce disagreements involving those who are part of the decision making process. In a study of 16 hospitals, Proctor and colleagues (1993) identified ethical dilemmas for social workers in 14% of the 395 cases examined. In more than half of the cases where ethical issues were present the conflict was over the client making decisions not considered to be in their best interests. In these situations the social workers were torn between commitment to client self-determination and concern that the patient was unable to assess their own needs accurately.

Another major category of ethical problems for this sample involved disagreements over discharge destination. Other areas of conflict for social workers were situations in which there were conflicts between the patient and family members or between patient and other hospital staff. It is important to note that the findings from this study were that the presence of ethical dilemmas were associated with delays in discharge and longer length of patient stay.

Abramson and associates (1993) reviewed two studies which evaluated disagreements in discharge planning. They found that 'disagreements occurred in at least one third of the cases, with most disagreements involving family members' (Abramson et al., 1993, p. 57). In both studies the level of disagreement among the hospital staff was low, but hospital staff were involved in disagreements with patients and with family members. Social workers also disagreed with patients. Both of these studies collected data from social workers rather than from patients. The position taken in their presentation was that disagreements are inevitable given the pressures involved in acute hospital care and that the existence of disagreements does not indicate dysfunction within the individual patient or family. It is important to understand the process of disagreements, the impact on patients and how social workers respond.

Whereas there are difficulties involved in obtaining data from patients about their disagreements with family or hospital staff it is essential to pursue information from the patients themselves. Clemens (1995) found differences in the perceptions of planners and family caregivers with regard to the decision making process. Family caregivers saw the hospital staff as coercing patients into nursing homes. The hospital staff were found to overrate the degree of patient and family influence over the process.

Social work productivity and cost drivers

Social work productivity studies

In a service industry like social work the use of resources is predominantly a matter of use of social workers' time. The major expenditures for social work intervention are the salaries paid to the social workers and social work administrators. Thus, the studies of social work productivity have focused on identification of factors that contribute to increased social work time expenditure.

The literature reviewed to date has not included recent cost accounting analysis of social work productivity although there have been studies of costs in the human services sector (Carr, 1993; Cooper and Kaplan, 1991; King, Lapsley, Mitchell, and Moyes, 1994) as well as analysis of pricing of health services within managed care (Kirk, 1995). There is a history of cost analysis in a few selected social work agencies (Hill, 1960) but the studies described were undertaken in the 1950's and the methods used were based on traditional cost accounting procedures. Within such traditional cost accounting procedures social work, as a labour intensive service, would be costed on the basis of standard rates of labour costs per hour with application of overhead per social work hour (Deakin and Maher, 1991). This approach has been adopted by those who have studied social work productivity in hospital settings (Spano and Lund, 1986; Volland, 1980).

The findings of social work productivity studies to date indicate that patient's length of stay and the number of problems experienced by the patients are associated with use of social work time (Coulton et al., 1985; Semke et al., 1993; Spano and Lund, 1986). Risk factors and types of problems have not emerged as factors which differentiate increased use of social work time in intervention in these studies. Coulton and associates (1985) found that, taken alone, the patient's number of problems was the strongest predictor of time utilisation, but that some types of intervention, namely discharge planning and psychosocial intervention, were also associated with increased use of social work time. The number of problems was also identified as associated with increased social work time expenditure by Spano and Lund (1986) and Semke and colleagues (1993).

Biopsychosocial functioning (internal and external resources in areas of self care, economics, cognitive, emotional, social and physical) also contributed to variation in use of social work services in the Coulton study (Coulton et al., 1985) but to a lesser degree than the number of problems. The study in a psychiatric unit of a tertiary care teaching hospital (Semke et al., 1993) found that Asian background, referral to child protection services and services to Medicaid patients in need of placement in a structured living environment, were associated with higher usage of social work time.

Within social work productivity studies the translation of social work time into dollar equivalent amounts has rarely been done except for administrative purposes (Hill, 1960; Spano and Lund, 1986). Whereas in the 1980's there were attempts to develop systems to measure the costs of social work services (Haber-Scharf, 1985; Volland, 1980) the current framework provided by the Society for Social Work Administrators in Health Care (Keller et al., 1993) emphasises measurement of social work time only. Where the translation to dollar terms has been done there has usually been reliance on a standard cost per social work hour based on total social work salary budget or some variation of that (Spano and Lund, 1986). The extensive costing of all aspects of service provision conducted by Knapp (Knapp et al., 1990) in relation to community based mental health services in Britain has not been pursued in relation to social work intervention in hospital settings.

Neither has there been application of cost accounting procedures. From the social work point of view standard costing may be considered an arbitrary process that does not take into account the complexities of social work service delivery. With standard costing the costs which vary according to how much service is provided, variable costs, would be defined as an amount per hour of social work time devoted to service delivery and all other costs (e.g. costs of equipment, training, administrative activities) would be treated as fixed costs. An average amount of fixed costs would be allocated per hour of social work service delivery time in order to define the total cost per hour of social work service (Deakin and Maher, 1991).

The relevance of this type of cost accounting procedure may have seemed marginal to social work in the past. With the predominance of salary costs in social work department budgets it has seemed easier to take a standard salary cost per social work hour as the basis for cost analysis than to bother with identification of which aspects of work tasks consume more resources. The complexities of cost accounting have been identified as too complex for human services (Vinter and Kish, 1984) and management accounting systems have been described as not providing information that is usable by line managers in human services (Hairston, 1985). The exception to this is the review of early efforts toward cost analysis in social welfare agencies which not only described attempts to develop analysis in relation to production and service centers but also included reports of detailed recording of social work activities and time allocated to the different activities (Hill, 1960).

The current form of activity costing (Cooper and Kaplan, 1991) provides a more usable and potentially helpful framework for analysis of costs in relation to social work activity. In activity based costing the costs are traced from work activities to products or services to establish the causal links between the activities which use resources and the outputs produced. The cost may be examined through levels of analysis. The levels defined by Cooper (1990) are:

- unit level activities (activities that are directly connected to the production of the service, e.g. search amongst alternatives for housing or placement for a patient);

- batch level activities (activities that are performed in relation to a group of services and which cannot be divided per unit of service, e.g. team meeting to discuss all patients in a ward);

- product level activities (activities that are related to a particular product/service, e.g. training in family therapy techniques);

- facility level activities (activities which sustain the process of providing services e.g. receptionist services).

By using these levels of activities as a framework or through analysis of the steps in the process of social work intervention it is possible to trace costs associated with different social work services and different client groups. The activity based framework is explicit and it is one which can account for complexities in provision of services through examination of a number of cost drivers which influence use of resources. To apply this to social work activity there would need to be an examination of social work time beyond the recording of time spent with patients. The time spent in supervision and training which could be traced to particular kinds of services or particular patients would need to be recorded. There also needs to be identification of the major cost drivers and this task has not yet been completed for social work in health care settings. The key to development of an accurate costing system is the selection of cost drivers which influence the flow of costs.

Cost drivers

From the social work productivity studies (Coulton et al., 1985; Semke et al., 1993) the indications are that number of problems and length of stay in hospital are two potential cost drivers in relation to social work intervention. Because of the findings in the study of the psychiatric unit (Semke et al., 1993) ethnicity should be added to the list. That study identified Asian background as significantly associated with increased use of social work resources. This finding implies that because of cultural or language difficulties, or due to the nature of the problems experienced by patients of Asian background more social work time is required than is the case for patients from other ethnic backgrounds (Semke et al., 1993). However, other findings from these two studies do not give any indication as to what characteristics of patients might be associated with a high level of demand on social work time and subsequent higher costs.

In relation to medical services Ramsey (1994) suggests that length of stay constitutes cycle time in the production of services and is therefore an important cost driver. He also proposes that levels of acuity may also differentiate which patients require more costly services. The problem with accepting that length of stay is a central cost driver for social work intervention is that the patients do not stay in hospital because of high levels of psychosocial acuity. There should be something more definitive about patients than the seriousness of their medical condition and number of problems they experience which influences how much social work service they utilise. Further exploration of cost drivers is a necessary preliminary step to application of activity based costing to social work intervention in a hospital setting. Because disagreements occur to a considerable extent in the social work patient populations (Abramson et al., 1993) and because disagreements may be seen as likely to add to the discomfort for patients it may be considered a potential cost driver.

2 A framework for analysis of decisions and disagreements

The current pressures contained within the health care system impose on social workers a need to ensure that the patient has control over decisions which affect their lives. Much of the literature on decision making within social work has focused on the social worker's decisions (Cuzzi et al., 1993) but the conceptual structures may be used to study decision making from the patient's perspective as shown by the Coulton studies (Coulton et al., 1988; Coulton et al., 1989).

Decision making and disagreements from the patient's perspective

The definition of six aspects of decision making by Coulton and colleagues (Coulton et al., 1988) provides a framework for analysis of the characteristics and barriers to decision making. The emphasis in these six aspects is on whether the patient has sufficient time, information, support and freedom from pressure and anxiety to promote effective decision making. Three of the scales, certainty about outcomes, control over decisions and family support, might be described as representing aspects which facilitate decision making. The other three, hypervigilance, restricted choice and time pressure or rushed decision making, may be identified as inhibitors to decision making.

The family support factor of the six decision making aspects deals with whether the family supports or takes over the decision making. The control factor concerns whether the patient is able to make the decision or have influence over the decision. The certainty factor deals with 'whether the outcome of the decision is knowable and understandable' (Coulton et al., 1988, p. 220) and incorporates whether the patient has sufficient information for decision making. The rushed factor is about time to decide.

In defining disagreements between patients and hospital staff there are specific areas which might be expected to provoke differences of opinion. Because of the pressures to discharge patients quickly it may be anticipated that there may be disagreements about the timing of discharge (Abramson, 1990; Brown and Furstenberg, 1992) and where the patient may be sent from the hospital (Coulton, 1990; Reinhardy, 1995). The other major area where disagreements may be anticipated is in relation to the treatment received or planned (Proctor et al., 1993). These same issues may be part of disagreements between patients and their family and in addition there are the problems which might arise from the impact of the patient's illness on family roles and responsibilities (Abramson et. al., 1993).

It is proposed that limitations on decision making by the patient, including disagreements, affect the outcomes for the patient and the amount of time the social worker must devote to the patient and family. The relationship between aspects of decision making and outcomes is presented in Figure 1. The facilitators of certainty about outcomes, control over decisions and family support are seen as assisting the decision making process so that patients feel less stress and are able to deal with the adjustments to the illness and other problems which arise more easily. The inhibitors to decision making, the anxiety, restricted choice and time pressure, as well as disagreements are seen as impediments to decision making increasing the level of difficulty and adding to the problems experienced by the patient. These barriers to patient decision making are also hypothesised to be associated with poorer outcomes for the patient in terms of reduction in problems and satisfaction with decisions as perceived by the patient. The six decision making scales are supplemented by the disagreements that may be part of a decision making situation. Disagreements may be defined 'as conflicts among the participants' (Abramson et al., 1993, p. 61) as perceived by the patient. That is, if

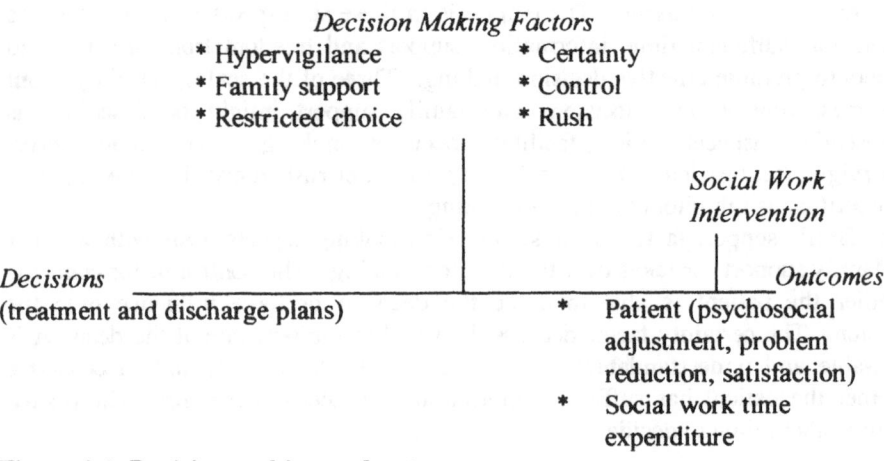

Figure 2.1 Decision making and outcomes

16

the patient does not perceive a conflict between themselves and family or hospital staff then a state of disagreement does not exist.

In addition it is proposed that the same limitations on decision making by the patient have an impact on the social work intervention. It is suggested that where there is inhibition to the decision making process and when disagreements occur the social work intervention takes more time, including time in direct work with patient and family, time in consultation with hospital colleagues and time in supervision.

Although there is debate as to whether it is possible to identify a generalised trait such as having an internal or external locus of control (Ajzen, 1991) it is considered possible that there may be individual differences between patients in terms of whether the patient expects to have control over decisions (Coulton et al., 1989). To assess this, a separate measure of locus of control might be considered appropriate. However, this study focuses on the limitations on decision making and the existence of disagreements as defined by the patient. If the patient expects to have little control over decisions then that patient is not likely to identify a lack of decision making opportunity. In other words, the patient will define whether the decision situation deprived them of an opportunity to make choices and this will account for individual differences in locus of control.

It is also clear that in this model there is no measurement of family disagreement with the hospital system although such conflicts have been identified as occurring frequently (Abramson et al., 1993). In this study the focus is on the patient's perceptions and outcomes.

Outcomes from the patients' perspective

Patient satisfaction

Patient satisfaction with services given is often used as a measure of the quality of services (Patti, 1987). Within the health industry there have been ongoing studies of patient satisfaction (Cleary et al., 1991; Marshall, Hays, and Mazel, 1996; Ware, Wright, Snyder, and Chu, 1975) and there have also been specific studies of patient satisfaction with social work services (Garber, Brenner, and Litwin, 1986; Proctor et al., 1992) as well as studies which focus on particular aspects of services (Greenley and Schoenherr, 1981; Reinhardy, 1995). In health services satisfaction studies there is a general trend towards positive findings (Garber et al., 1986: Proctor et al., 1992). Most patients or clients described in these studies report that they are pleased with the services offered. However, people in poorer health may report higher levels of dissatisfaction (Cleary et al., 1991; Proctor et al., 1992) and age and income level are other factors which have been shown to affect satisfaction (Cleary et al., 1991). The analysis of a national telephone survey identified lower income and younger age as associated with higher reported problem scores (Cleary

17

et al., 1991). In a more recent study of the relationship between physical health status and mental health status with satisfaction with care there was an indication that mental health, rather than physical health, may have an influence on satisfaction ratings (Marshall et al., 1996). This particular study used structural equation modeling to examine the relationships and the authors concluded that further study of these relationships was required. Whether the decision making environment influences the level of satisfaction with decisions made has not been examined in any study reviewed to date.

Outcomes of social work intervention

As indicated by the recent study of ethical dilemmas (Proctor et al., 1993) there may well be debate as to what constitutes effective outcomes of social work intervention. The patient's wishes and choices may be seen as unwise or as potentially detrimental to the individual's well-being. However, given the lack of consensus about what the right outcomes may be, there is a strong justification for reliance on patient assessment of outcomes in situations where patients are mentally competent and able to determine what suits them best. To rely on the client's determination of outcomes achieved is in keeping with the Code of Ethics (NASW, 1990) and the principle of self-determination.

Given the short term intervention in a context where the patient and family may be in a crisis situation it is appropriate to define social work intervention as primarily directed toward problem solving and with the general goal of problem reduction. The outcomes then may be assessed in terms of the patient's perception of reduction in problems. While hospital admission has health problems as the primary focus for intervention, the social worker attends to a broad range of life domains which may be affected by the illness or treatment. Taking the productivity measurement system for social work in health care (Keller et al., 1993) as the guide, the major areas of problems may be defined as follows:

- Patient's living situation: adequacy of accommodation

- Financial issues

- Adjustment to illness and treatment

- Family adjustment to illness and treatment

- Family conflict

- Other family/relationship problems

18

- Emotional problems

- Employment/education problems

- Legal problems

Social work time expenditure and cost drivers

In the absence of defined time requirements for different social work interventions measurement of social work time must rely on social work records of time allocated to patients. Observation and time sampling of social workers activities would not allow measurement of time expenditure in relation to a large number of patients and so the source for information must be the records kept by social workers. Time allocated to patients includes time spent in interviews with patients and families, in preparation for and making records of interviews, in follow-up actions on behalf of patients and families, and in consultation with other staff about patients.

The potential cost drivers include patient length of stay and the number and type of problems, patient ethnicity, and the presence of disagreement in the patient's decision making system.

Hypotheses

On the basis of the literature review the study hypotheses are:

- Patients who perceive their decision making as involving higher family support, certainty about the future, and control over choices will have a higher level of satisfaction with decisions made while in hospital.

- Family support, certainty about the future, and control over choices in decision making are positively associated with positive psychosocial outcomes.

- The association between the negative aspects of decision making (hypervigilance, disagreements, restricted choices and little time) and negative psychosocial outcomes for the patient decrease substantially for patients who received social work intervention.

- The patient's experience of disagreements in decision making, the number and type of problems experienced by the patient, the patient's ethnicity, and length of stay in hospital are related to higher use of social work resources.

3 Research design and methodology

Study design

This study has two sections both of which were designed in the form of cross sectional survey procedures. The first part is an examination of the nature of decision making experienced by a sample of social work and non social work hospital patients from one acute care teaching hospital in Boston. The second part is an examination of the utilisation of resources by the social work sample. The data collected included responses to post discharge telephone interviews, information supplied by social workers and data collected from computerised documents.

Part 1

For the study of decision making processes during hospitalisation data collection had to be completed after the hospital treatment and discharge. No pretests could be completed prior to hospitalisation as admission to hospital was not necessarily a predictable event.

The patients were randomly selected from discharge lists but they were not randomly allocated to the two groups: social work and non social work. Since the patients in both groups were patients in the same hospital during a three month period they may be considered cohorts which provide quasi comparability of groups. A random sample of non social work patients was decided on instead of a matched group in order to prevent the matching process interfering with data analysis (Campbell and Stanley, 1963). Campbell and Stanley (1963) outline the possibility that the variables on which patients are matched may be correlated with exposure to the treatment and thus will affect the measurement of the observation.

Indeed, this may apply in this context. For example, if non social work patients had been matched to social work patients on the basis of illness, age and ethnicity there may have been some confusion in the analysis. There may well be some differentiation in referrals to social work on the basis of these variables which would affect measures taken in the post discharge period.

Part 2

For the second part of the study, data for the social work group only was designated for analysis and the cross sectional data about resources utilised was collected retrospectively. That is, details of social work resource utilisation was derived from computerised documents after social work intervention had been completed.

Sampling

The hospital in which this study was based is a 750 bed teaching hospital providing a variety of specialist medical and surgical services to a widely diverse population in Boston. The social work department has 40 social workers who provide services to some community projects as well as to inpatients and outpatients of the hospital. During 1994 the hospital provided services to 36,498 inpatients and the social work department provided services to 5,956 of these patients. In 1995, the year of the study, the hospital provided services to 35,443 patients. From these figures it is estimated that social work services were provided to approximately 5,600 during 1995.

Like all acute hospitals this medical center receives only the most seriously ill patients as inpatients and in spite of serious medical conditions most patients stay in the hospital for very short periods of time. Therefore, only patients who had a length of stay of three days or more were included in the study. The exception to this was for obstetrics patients. For this group of patients a length of stay of 2 days or more was considered sufficient to include them in the sample. Social workers advised that exclusion of obstetrics patients admitted for less than 3 days would mean that this substantial part of the hospital population would not be represented adequately.

Selection procedures

The sample for the study was obtained through stratified random sampling of the population of patients discharged from the hospital between April and June 1995. The sample consisted of patients seen by a social worker (SW) and patients not seen by a social worker (NSW). These two groups were selected independently and randomly.

For the social work sample the social work department registration system provided the population. Lists of patients registered as receiving social work services were extracted from the computerised recording system for each week of the study duration. Fifty patients were then selected using a table of random numbers (Frankfort-Nachmias and Nachmias, 1992). The hospital computerised information system was then consulted to obtain basic information about the patients (see Appendix A). At this point the following patients were eliminated from the study: those who were listed as deceased, did not have a telephone number recorded, had been admitted for less than the required length of stay, did not live in New England, were non English speaking, or who were listed as having restricted files. Patients who had been randomly selected but who had been re admitted remained in the sample.

A comparison group of patients who did not receive social work services during hospitalisation in the same time period were randomly selected from hospital discharge lists. This list was in the form of a special report produced for this study. The list included details of medical record number, discharge date and Diagnostic Related Group (DRG) code for each patient (Kasten, 1986) . The selection process was the same as for the social work sample except that the non social work patients were selected from only two lists of patients discharged between April/ May and May/ June 1995. The hospital was not able to produce discharge lists week by week for this group.

After selection, patients were sent letters which invited them to participate in the study (Appendix B). Enclosed with the letter was a reply card which allowed patients to decline participation in the study (Appendix B). In addition, the telephone number for the social work department was provided so that potential respondents could contact the Director of Social Work for further information if they wished to do so.

Two weeks after mailing the letters the patients were telephoned to reconfirm their willingness to participate. During the first telephone contact any questions about the study were answered and times were arranged for the interview. Some patients requested that the interview be completed at the time of the first call. This was done if at all possible. When this did not occur, telephone interviews were scheduled for a time that was convenient for the respondents.

The sample characteristics

The total number of patients who were selected and sent letters was 582. A total of 196 patients were interviewed including 96 social work patients (SW) and 100 non social work patients (NSW). The response rate in relation to the original letters of invitation was 34%.

Almost half of the group not interviewed (48.2%) gave no reason or simply stated they did not wish to be involved. Only 63 (16%) of the 386 people not interviewed returned the card to indicate that they did not wish to be involved. Some of the

23

most frequently mentioned reasons for not participating included patients who were too ill or not mentally competent, some who had already participated in a survey from the same hospital, and a few people who could not speak English. There were also a number who had died and quite a large group who had moved, were away on holiday or who had changed their telephone number. Some of the group not located may have died, moved to other addresses, or may have been re admitted to the hospital.

To some extent the high attrition rate in this seriously ill population was expected. However, 40% of those not interviewed were people who could not participate because they could not communicate and they should not have been selected into the sample. It is the fifty percent of those not interviewed who made clear decisions not to be part of the study who might be more accurately described as non responders within the total sample. This group presents a risk of unknown bias in the results.

It was not anticipated that there would be a difference in the response rate between social work and non social patient groups. Sixty-six percent of non social work patients and 41% of social work patients agreed to be interviewed. A higher proportion of social work patients were too ill to be interviewed (SW 17.4% compared with NSW 7.3%) or not mentally competent (SW 7.2% compared with NSW 2%). More social work patients had died after leaving hospital (SW 5.5% compared with NSW 3.3%).

Other comparisons show few differences between the social work and non social work groups. In terms of geographical location as shown by the zip codes the largest number of people lived in Massachusetts (90.5%) and most of those resided in Boston (47.2% of the total sample). The largest group from another state was the 26 (4.5%) from New Hampshire. There appears to be similar numbers across different geographic areas for both social work patients and non social work patients.

Fifty-four percent of the sample were married or with partners, 23% were single, 11% widowed and 9% separated or divorced. These proportions appear to be consistent across the social work patients and non social work patients interviewed. For the non interviewed patients there are variations in the proportions of those separated or widowed when compared with the group who were interviewed, but the predominance of married people is consistent across both the social work and non social work groups. The social work sample has a higher proportion of widowed people among those not interviewed.

In the total group of 582 patients 63% were female and 37% male. Similar proportions are found in both the interviewed and non interviewed groups. These proportions parallel those for the total patient population of the hospital in 1995 (64% female, 36% male). In the non interviewed non social work group there was a slightly larger proportion of males (44%).

The known characteristics of the patients selected into the sample were examined to explore whether there were any specific factors which made it more likely that a patient, once selected, would be interviewed. The question is, were there factors that influenced whether patients were interviewed or not? Bivariate tests of association were carried out in relation to whether patient category, patient's medical unit, patient's gender, patient's marital status or patient's geographical location were associated with being interviewed. The chi square results were not significant in examination of the association between gender or marital status and being interviewed. Both patient's medical unit (X^2 = 34.85, df = 18, p < .01; Lambda = .01) and patient's geographical location (X^2= 24.32, df = 11, p < .05; Lambda = .01) produced significant chi square results. The lambda coefficient was very small indicating that these variables are independent. The implication is that there was a difference in chances of being interviewed according to which medical unit the patient was admitted but this was not a strong indicator as to whether any individual might be interviewed. Similarly, being from particular areas in New England was associated with the chance of being interviewed but again this was not a strong indicator.

The chi square in relation to being a social work or non social work patient and being interviewed was significant (X^2 = 7.51, df = 1, p < .01). The lambda for this association produced a zero correlation (Lambda = .000). As noted by Pilcher (1990) this sometimes occurs even when there is some degree of correlation. In those circumstances the best indication of the level of correlation may be obtained from the other measures. The Uncertainty Coefficient (Uncertainty Coefficient = .01), the proportion of uncertainty in the dependent variable reduced by information about the independent variable, produced a coefficient of .01 and this indicates that these variables, patient category (social work or not social work) and being interviewed, are independent.

A final question considered was whether there were significant differences between the social work and non social work samples in relation to the known characteristics of both groups. The question was whether patient's gender, marital status, medical unit, geographical location, and reasons for not being interviewed were significantly associated with being a social work versus a non social work patient.

Both gender and geographical location showed no significant results. There was no increased chance of being a social work patient associated with gender or home address. Marital status (X^2 = 14.85, df = 3, p < .01; Lambda = .000 Uncertainty Coefficient = .01), patients medical unit (X^2 = 86.04, df = 18, p < .001; Lambda = .21), and reason for not being interviewed (X^2 = 20.18, df = 8, p < .01; Lambda = .03) all produced significant results. The moderate Lambda coefficient related to the patient's medical unit (Lambda = .21) is the coefficient with patient category as social work or non social work as the dependent variable. As a PRE measure it indicates that that there is a 21% reduction in error in predicting which patients in this sample would be seen by social workers given information about to which medical category the patient belonged (Norusis, 1993; Pilcher, 1990). This is not surprising given that in most teaching hospitals social work departments allocate staff to medical units where there is an expectation that the nature of the medical condition will be associated with increased problems for the patients and their families. The Lambda and Uncertainty Coefficient results for marital status and reason for not being interviewed were very low and so while there is an association between these variables (marital status, reason for not being interviewed) and being a social work or non social work patient it is not a strong indicator. That is, knowing a patient's reason for not being interviewed or their marital status would not reduce much error in predicting which patients might be seen by a social worker during their stay in the hospital.

Issues arising from sampling

To the extent that information about the non interviewed patients was available the comparisons of the two selected samples indicates that there are some differences between the two groups. The chi square results taken together indicate that it is reasonable to assume that the variables examined were not strong and significant factors of bias in the selection of the sample in most instances. The exception to this is that social work patients and non social work patients may well have been drawn from different medical unit populations in the hospital since the association between patient category and medical unit produced a moderate and significant association. While this may have influenced the results, examination of the impact of medical condition or medical unit would require a separate study. The focus for the current research was on the decision making environment and resource utilisation of a broad cross section of the hospital population and did not include any attempt to examine the impact of particular disease and recovery processes. Information about patients' ethnicity was not collected during the sampling process and therefore no analysis of the influence of ethnicity is possible.

The most important aspect of analysis of the sample is that there was a high attrition rate and that social work patients were less likely to be interviewed than non social work patients. The high attrition rate, with approximately half of the non respondents making a decision not to participate, meant that two thirds of the total group contacted was lost. Response rates of 70% to 80% may be considered the norm for social surveys (Moser and Kalton, 1971) so this loss of two thirds of the original sample constitutes a very high attrition rate. It is known that telephone surveys may have higher refusal rates than face-to-face interviews (Marcus and Telesky, 1983). The responses from the large group of non responders may have had a substantial impact on the findings.

The low response rate, particularly from social work patients, means that there is a need for caution in generalisation of findings even to the hospital population at the time of the study.

Measurement

The telephone interviews with social work and non social work patients were the primary source of data for the first part of the study which was devoted to decision making. Additional data was taken from the Social Work Department computerised statistics system and from information supplied by social workers, and these sources provided the data for the second part of the study which focused on resource utilisation.

Part 1: Decision making

The Telephone Interview Schedule includes questions in the following areas (Appendix C contains the Interview Schedule):

Independent variables

Decision making facilitating variables: family support, certainty and control. The facilitator variables, *family support, certainty*, and control were measured by three subscales of the decision making scale developed by Coulton et al. (1988). These questions were answered using a five point scale: not at all true, somewhat true, half true and half false, mostly true and completely true. The family support scale included questions 14 to 16, which asked questions about the degree to which the patient felt that family members supported the patient's thinking and decision making. The certainty scale included questions 20 to 23, which asked about the extent to which the patient had felt certain about how they would fare after leaving the hospital, about whether the patient had sufficient information, and whether the patient knew what the doctor thought the patient should decide. Finally, the control scale included questions 24 and 25, which asked the patient to rate the degree to which they felt they had choice and final say about the decision.

These scales were validated by Coulton and her colleagues as a measure of patient decision making using a sample of 314 patients over the age of 60 years who were about to be discharged from a large, urban, university affiliated hospital. The reliability analysis in the Coulton study produced a reliability coefficient of .70 for the family support scale. The control scale produced an alpha coefficient of .62 and the certainty scale reached the .51 level only. Some of the low reliability levels may be due to the small number of items in the individual scales (Smith, 1975). Although there are warnings given about setting an acceptable standard for reliability (Pedhazur and Pedhazur-Schmelkin, 1991) it seems that .70 or .80 is

27

often cited as the benchmark (Fischer and Corcoran, 1994; Pedhazur and Pedhazur-Schmelkin, 1991). An enticing argument put forward (Pedhazur and Pedhazur-Schmelkin, 1991) is the proposal that Nunnally (1967) considered that for early stages of research a coefficient of .50 would suffice. However the conclusion seems to be that the amount of error considered acceptable must be the guide (Pedhazur and Pedhazur-Schmelkin, 1991). In this instance the reliability for the certainty scale is below the acceptable level.

Decision making inhibitor factors: hypervigilance, restricted choice and being rushed. The inhibitor variables of *hypervigilance, restricted choice and being rushed* were measured by three subscales of the decision making scale developed by Coulton et al. (1988). These questions were answered using a five point scale: not at all true, somewhat true, half true and half false, mostly true and completely true. The hypervigilance scale included questions 7 to 13. These questions asked the patient to rate the degree to which they felt that their situation when they were in the hospital was hopeless, whether they had worried or fearful about what would happen to them after leaving hospital, and whether they felt that everyone was trying to tell them what to do. The restricted choice scale included questions 17 to 19, which asked questions about the degree to which the patient experienced having choices to make and whether the decisions they made appeared to be final ones. The rushed scale included questions 26 and 27, which asked questions about perceptions of being rushed in making decisions while they were in the hospital.

As in the case of the decision making facilitator scales, these inhibitor scales were validated by Coulton and her colleagues as a measure of patient decision making using a sample of 314 patients over the age of 60 years who were about to be discharged from a large, urban, university affiliated hospital. The reliability analysis in the Coulton study produced a reliability coefficient of .75 for the hypervigilance scale. The restricted choice scale produced an alpha coefficient .60 while the rushed scale reached the .51 level only. As stated earlier the low reliability coefficients may be related to the small number of items in the scales and the reliability coefficients for both the rushed scale and the restricted choice scale are not acceptable if the benchmark of .70 is taken as the required level.

However, taken overall the results in relation to the decision making scales may be considered acceptable if not ideal for an exploratory study. These scales appear the most well constructed and validated measures available that relate to patient decision making in the hospital context, especially when the search is for a measure which incorporates patient and family interaction in decision making as well as the patient and health provider perspective (Coulton, 1990).

Disagreements in decision making. The questions on patient's perceptions of disagreements in decision making were developed for this study. They asked patients to identify whether or not they had experienced disagreements in the specified areas. The categories developed for examination of disagreements were derived from the literature on discharge planning and from an understanding of issues which arise for patients which has been developed over years of social work practice. It was expected that disagreements with hospital staff may be about treatment plans or treatment that had already been given as well as in relation to discharge arrangements. In relation to the questions about family disagreements the questions were focused on the issues which might arise as part of the treatment process as well as those which may occur because of patient's absence from the family home.

It was not anticipated that patients would feel a need to respond in any particular direction. It was expected that there would be individual differences as to whether patients view disagreements as positive or negative events. That is, some patients may feel that it is acceptable to have disagreements with hospital staff and others may not.

A total number of disagreements was calculated for each patient in relation to both disagreements with hospital staff and disagreements with family. Each of the questions about disagreements were in binary form, coded 0 for no disagreement and 1 to indicate that there had been some disagreement. Each 'yes' response to the question 'did you have a disagreement about' was scored as 1 point toward the total disagreement score. In both disagreements with hospital staff and disagreements with family there were seven areas of potential disagreement, and therefore, the highest possible disagreement score for any patient was seven.

Dependent variables

Patient satisfaction with decision making. The single question asking patients how satisfied they were with decisions they made while they were in the hospital constitutes one of the outcome measures. The inadequacies of a global question are acknowledged but there appeared to be no alternative brief measure of how well satisfied patients felt about the way decisions were made. The simple question appeared appropriate.

Problems scale. This was the outcome measure. The nine categories of problems rated by patients were taken from the productivity measurement system devised for social work administration in health care settings (Keller et al., 1993). The categories were accommodation, financial, adjustment to illness, family adjustment to the illness, family relationships, other relationships, emotional, school or work and legal problems. Respondents were able to identify other problems if they wished to do so. They were asked to rate the problems they had at the time of the interview. They were also asked to report on problems they had while in the hospital. A final component requested that they identify who helped them with each of the problems they experienced while they were in the hospital. The choices given to them about who had helped them included doctors, nurses, social workers, family members, no one or other people. They were also able to respond that help was not needed.

This type of post/then questioning which asks people to reflect on the past has been used with good results in the context of educational programs and in a test of General Well-Being (Doueck and Bondanza, 1990; Howard, 1980; Nicholson, Belcastro, and Gold, 1985). The benefits of a retrospective test appear to be the control of a form of response-shift bias which may distort comparisons of pre and post test measures. For example, in the context of pre and post tests to measure effectiveness of a training program participants may claim more knowledge than they possess when completing the pre test. By giving two tests at the end of the training -- one which asks what they know at the end of the training and the other which asks what they knew before the training -- a more accurate measure is said to be obtained. In these studies the retrospective responses, where subjects reflect on what they experienced at a point in time in the past, have been presented as a valid substitute for the pretest. It is as a substitute for a pre test measure that the post/then questions were included in this context.

The use of post/then measures has been criticised by Pedhazur and Pedhazur-Schmelkin (1991) because the procedure is expected to introduce additional sources of error to measurement of change processes because of factors such as respondents forgetting or becoming confused about what happened in the past. The limitations of the post/then approach were accepted but it was decided to use it as the best available alternative in a situation where pre tests could not easily be obtained for a large sample of patients.

Control variables

Demographic characteristics. Details of patients' demographic characteristics were included in the questionnaire schedule and in the data collected from hospital information systems. The information collected included details of age, gender, and marital status. Patients were asked to indicate which category they belonged to in relation to ethnicity and level of annual income for their household (Appendix C). In addition to the level of household income, patients were asked for the number of years of education they had completed as a second measure of socioeconomic status.

Because of the nature of the population of this sample the ethnicity variable could only be used as a binary variable with 1 indicating that the patient was white and 0 indicating that the patient was not white. While there was a substantial number of African-American patients in the study group there were very few people of Asian, Hispanic or any other ethnic origin. Similarly, more than half of the sample were married or living in a stable relationship so that variable was also used as a binary variable with 1 indicating that the patient was married and 0 indicating that the patient was not married.

Characteristics of the patients' stay in the hospital. The form for collection of information from the computerised hospital information system is presented in Appendix A. The primary purpose of this information was to obtain accurate details of patient length of stay in hospital and to obtain a medical code to the patient's diagnosis so that both of these variables might be included as control variables. In addition, information about the gap between the patient's date of discharge and the date of interview was also recorded. Both length of stay and the gap between discharge and interview were recorded in terms of number of days.

No test of the reliability of the hospital information system was carried out and it is not known whether any system exists for auditing the system's integrity in data entry.

Final open ended questions

The final questions were designed to allow patients to provide responses in their own words. The first question obtained an overall response from the patient about their perception of control in decision making. The second asked patients about the impact of disagreements on their decision making and planning for the future. While the questions allowed patients to describe their experiences in their own words, the questions about the control they had and the disagreements they experienced were also coded as yes/no responses. An additional question allowed respondents to add information if they wished to do so.

Part 2: Resource utilisation

Costing of social work intervention. Costing of social work time expenditure for each social work patient in the study was done on the basis of hourly salary rates obtained for each worker in the study. Details of additional salary costs for supervisors were also obtained.

Details of time expenditure were collected from the departmental computerised statistics systems and from additional information supplied by the social workers (Appendix A).

An interview with the Director of Social Work identified that the only routinely provided social work service supplied to patients by the hospital was subsidised parking. The parking fees subsidy register was consulted to extract details of the subsidies given to study patients and their families. It was not possible to obtain information about the total departmental expenditures in order to do comparison of costing from traditional costing and activity based costing perspectives.

The information obtained during the study provided details of:

- social work time in service delivery to each patient,

- supervision, training and any other time expenditure,

- salary costs per social worker and per social work supervisor, on costs per social worker,

- parking subsidy provided to each patient and their family, and

- details of any other expenditures provided for the patient and family by the social worker.

In summary, the data obtained allowed for retrospective product costing per patient excluding fixed costs. Details of the fixed costs of department accommodation and utilities, computer services, administration and reception services, general training budget and other consumables were not made available.

Statistical analysis

Part 1: Decision making - Computations of scales and outcome scores

Decision making scales. Scores were computed for the decision making sub scales, and for usefulness of social work/hospital staff member interventions. For the decision making scales the scoring procedure involved summing the item values and dividing by the number of items (Coulton et al., 1988). The scales were examined for approximation to normal distribution, submitted to orthogonal factor analysis and internal consistency analysis using Cronbach's alpha.

Problem scores. The ratings made by patients were summed to form a *problems now* (sum of scores of problems at the time of interview) and *problems then* (sum of scores of problems when in the hospital) score. In each case the highest possible score was 60. For the post/then calculation a problem difference score was calculated by subtracting the problems now scores from the problems then scores.

Other variables. Two additional variables included in the analysis were *length of patient* stay in the hospital and the *gap* between discharge and interview dates. These were calculated in the form of number of days.

Multiple regression analysis

All analyses for comparability of the sub groups in the sample (social work and non social work) have been by multiple regression analysis. Multiple linear regression analysis consists of a process of analysing the linear variability of the dependent variable in relation to the specified independent variables. It allows for examination of the relationships between study variables and includes a capacity to control for the influence of other factors that may impinge on the relationships between the primary independent and dependent variables. This process enables the patient category variable (whether a patient had received social work services or not) to be included in a regression equation in order to examine whether being a social work patient affects the results. Regression analysis also allows for comparability of sub groups within the sample by inclusion of the category of group membership variable in the equation. Given the size of the sample and the research questions focused on examination of the relationships between a number of independent variables with individual dependent variables, multiple regression is the most appropriate mode of analysis.

Multiple regression analysis also provides a measure of the goodness of fit for the theoretical model. The squared multiple correlation provides an estimate of the amount of variance of the dependent variable explained by the set of independent variables. While simultaneous entry of variables into the equation is the recommended approach because it requires the specification of the theoretical structure prior to conducting the analysis (Pedhazur et al., 1991) it is also acceptable to use backward elimination methods in an exploratory study where the objective is to describe relationships between variables or where there is an attempt to define an equation which predicts the level of the dependent variable as accurately as possible (Afifi and Clark, 1990; Hair, Anderson, Tatham, and Black, 1995).

While Pedhazur and Pedhazur-Schmelkin (1991) present a strongly worded argument against any form of regression analysis other than simultaneous entry of the variables the acceptance by other authors indicates that sequential entry analysis may be used in an exploratory or model building phase of study. It is particularly useful in assisting the exploration of the contributions made to the difference in the squared multiple correlation by different combinations of variables. Although backward elimination is not 'expected to produce the best possible equation for a given number of variables to be included' (Afifi and Clark, 1990, p. 200) this procedure does reduce the number of variables to be considered so a concise model may be examined (Norusis, 1993). In this context it is necessary to explore the relationship between the independent variables and the dependent variable in each equation but it is also important to examine the contribution of other variables which may influence those relationships. Therefore, sequential regression analyses have been used in relation to all hypotheses.

Part 2: Resource utilisation

The cost for each patient was derived by summing the service delivery time, supervision time, training time and any other time expenditure identified by the social worker and this total time was multiplied by the rate per hour for the identified social worker to produce cost 1. The Director of Social Work advised that for each social worker there were additional costs such as insurance, leave and other unavoidable expenses incurred for each employee within the hospital. These expenses were identified as costing an additional 25% of each salary. Therefore, a second calculation was done multiplying cost 1 by the .25 rate for the usual additional costs to determine cost 2. Cost 1 and cost 2 were summed to produce cost 3. The supervision time was then multiplied by the hourly rate for the supervisor (cost 3) and a similar calculation for the usual additional costs for the supervisor's time was done (cost 4). Cost 3 and cost 4 were summed to provide the total cost of the supervisor's time as cost 6. The service delivery cost and the supervision cost were summed to form the total social work time cost identified as cost 7. Finally, the total case cost was calculated by adding cost 7 to the value of parking subsidies and any other expenses identified by social workers. The costs for interns who receive no salary was limited to costs of supervision, parking and other expenditures. While it was possible to calculate a standard cost of intern to the social work department this was not done as there was no allocation of fixed costs for the case costs for social work staff. To have included standardised costs for one part of the total group of social work practitioners would have introduced inconsistency of the basis for the costing.

The hypotheses related to analysis of cost drivers was also tested using sequential regression analysis. The task in identification of cost drivers is to establish which factors contribute to an increase in expenditure of resources. Therefore, sequential multiple linear regression analysis is appropriate because it allows examination of the contribution of the individual independent variables, the potential cost drivers, in accounting for the variance of the dependent variable, the cost of social work services. To obtain this data, stepwise regression analysis was chosen because the series of equations allow examination of different combinations of independent variables as variables are included or excluded in the sequential equations.

4 Results: Decision making

This chapter includes a description of the sample characteristics and the findings from statistical tests of the hypotheses related to patient decision making. Data analysis for the second part of the study, resource utilisation, appears in Chapter 6.

The major hypotheses in relation to patient decision making were as follows:

Hypothesis 1: Patients who perceive their decision making as involving more family support, certainty about the future, and control over choices will have a higher level of satisfaction with decisions made in the hospital than those who perceive their decision making as involving less family support, less certainty about the future, and less control over choices.

Hypothesis 2: Family support, certainty about the future, and control over choices in decision making are positively associated with positive psychosocial outcomes.

Hypothesis 3: The association between the negative aspects of decision making (hypervigilance, disagreements, restricted choices and little time) and unfavorable psychosocial outcomes for the patient decrease substantially for patients who received social work intervention.

Sample characteristics

Demographic characteristics

The demographic characteristics of respondents are presented in Table 4.1.

The group of patients in this sample were predominately older, married, female and white. Slightly more than half of the people interviewed were more than 50 years of age. There were few people of Asian, Hispanic/Latino or American Native Indian origin. The low number of Asian patients is consistent with the proportion of this group in the total hospital population for 1995. However, the sample has more American Indians than might be expected and fewer Hispanic people than might be expected.

This study collected data from patients who primarily lived with family members (77%) rather than alone (19%), with friends (2%), or in institutions (2%). The group of patients who were discharged to skilled nursing facilities or other long term residential care were not incorporated into the study. In terms of socioeconomic status this group of patients might be described as predominately educated and not poor. Ninety-four percent (94%) were high school graduates, 66% had attended college and 55% lived in households with an annual income of $30,000 or more. The homeless and poor were not well represented in this group of hospital patients.

In terms of age, gender, ethnicity, living arrangements and education levels the proportions were similar when social work and non social work groups were compared. The differences between the social work and non social work patients were in relation to marital status and income. In relation to marital status the major difference between the social work and non social work groups was the higher proportion of married women in the non social work group (66% of non social work women were married compared with 49% of social work women). There were more single women in the social work group (26% of social work women compared with 11% of non social work women).

In relation to income there were substantial differences between the social work and non social work groups. Forty-four percent (44%) of the social work patients interviewed reported incomes of $30,000 or less in comparison with 28% of the non social work patients. Twenty-eight percent (28%) of the non social work group fell into the higher middle income group ($50,000 to $69,999) compared with 8% of the social work group.

Clinical characteristics

The subjects in this study were from a broad cross section of hospital patients as shown by Table 4.2. The highest numbers of respondents were classified as having circulatory system (21%) or musculo-skeletal system disorders (18%). Another large group of patients were classified under female reproductive or pregnancy and related conditions (19%). There were more social work patients than non social work patients with disorders in the areas of nervous system, musculo-skeletal, skin and breast, kidney, and infectious diseases. There were higher numbers of non social work patients in categories of respiratory, circulatory, digestive system, hepatobiliary conditions, and pregnancy.

Table 4.1
Demographic characteristics of patients (n = 196)

Variable	Number	Percentage	
Age:			
18 - 49	92	47%	
50 - 69	70	36%	
70 - 89	34	17%	
Gender:			
Male	69	35%	
Female	127	65%	
Marital Status:			
Married	112	57%	
Single	38	19%	
Widowed	23	12%	
Separated/Divorced	23	12%	
Ethnicity:			*Hospital popn.*[a]
White	168	86%	70%
(European origin)			
Black	22	11%	15%
(African American and others)			
Native Indian	3	1%	.0005%
Asian-American	2	1%	.02%
(Asian)			
Hispanic/Latino	1	0%	.09%

table continues

Table 4.1 continued
Demographic characteristics of patients (n = 196)

Variable	Number	Percentage
Living Arrangement:		
With spouse and children	61	31%
With spouse or partner	50	25%
With children or other family	40	20%
Alone	37	19%
With friends	5	2%
Group living	3	1%
Household income: [b]		
Under $10,000	24	12%
$10,000 to $29,999	46	23%
$30,000 to $49,999	47	24%
$50,000 to $69,999	36	18%
$70,000 to 89,999	13	7%
$90,000 and over	11	6%
Education Level:		
Did not complete high school	12	6%
High school graduate	61	31%
Attended college	35	18%
College degree	42	21%
Postgraduate degree	46	23%
Total	196	100%

a.   Proportion of hospital patients in various categories of ethnicity for the year 1995

b.   Income data was not obtained from 19 patients.

Table 4.2
**Clinical characteristics of social work and
non social work patients (n = 196)**

Variable	SW n(%)	NSW n(%)	Total n(%)
Medical Diagnostic Category [a]			
Nervous system	8 (4%)	2 (1%)	10 (5%)
Ear, nose and throat	1 (0%)	1 (0%)	2 (1%)
Respiratory system	5 (3%)	10 (5%)	15 (8%)
Circulatory system	13 (7%)	28 (14%)	41 (21%)
Digestive system	1 (0%)	7 (4%)	8 (4%)
Hepatobiliary, pancreas	1 (0%)	5 (3%)	6 (3%)
Musculo-skeletal system	20 (10%)	15 (8%)	35 (18%)
Skin and breast	5 (2%)	1 (0%)	6 (3%)
Endocrine, nutritional	1 (0%)	1 (0%)	2 (1%)
Kidney and urinary tract	4 (2%)	1 (0%)	5 (2%)
Female reproductive	7 (3%)	7 (3%)	14 (7%)
Pregnancy and childbirth	10 (5%)	14 (7%)	24 (12%)
Blood and blood forming organs	1 (0%)	0 (0%)	1 (0%)
Infectious and parasitic diseases	11 (6%)	3 (1%)	14 (7%)
Injury, poisonings and drug toxicity	1 (0%)	2 (1%)	3 (1%)
Burns	1 (0%)	0 (0%)	1 (0%)
Other factors affecting health status	0 (0%)	1 (0%)	1 (0%)

table continues

Almost half of the total group of respondents were in the hospital for 5 days or less and 80% were in the hospital for less than 10 days. However, some longer stay patients were included in the sample. There appears to be no differences between social work and non social work patients in terms of length of stay for this sample of patients.

Table 4.2 continued
Clinical characteristics of social work and
non social work patients (n = 196)

Variable	SW n(%)	NSW n(%)	Total n(%)
Length of Stay:			
5 days and under	37 (19%)	47 (24%)	84 (43%)
6 to 10 days	37 (19%)	36 (18%)	73 (37%)
11 to 20 days	15 (8%)	14 (7%)	29 (15%)
21 to 30 days	6 (3%)	1 (0%)	7 (4%)
31 days or more	1 (0%)	2 (1%)	3 (1%)
Total	196 (49%)	100 (51%)	196 (100%)*

* Variation in total percentage due to rounding.

a. Medical Diagnostic category not obtained for 8 patients.

While the plan had been for patients to be interviewed approximately a month after discharge a number of factors interfered with this process. Some patients were readmitted to the hospital before the interview could take place. In addition, the sample for non social work patients was drawn from only two discharge lists instead of from weekly lists produced by the social work department. Because it was obvious that there was variation in when patients were interviewed in relation to their discharge date, the gap between discharge and interview in terms of days was recorded.

Social work patients were interviewed earlier after discharge than non social work patients. Most social work patients (86%) were interviewed within eight weeks of discharge, whereas 16% of non social work patients were interviewed later than two months. This data suggests that it is important to include this variable in the regression equations to examine whether the variation in timing of interviews had an influence on results obtained.

Decision making

Tests for normal distribution of decision making scales

The preliminary analysis of normal probability plots of the decision making scales revealed that none of the scales met the assumption of normal distribution. Each scale was examined for the potential to approximate normal distribution (Hair et al., 1995). The hypervigilance scale, the restricted choice scale and the rushed scale appeared likely to improve approximation to normal distribution through transformations. Natural log and square root transformations were completed and the results examined for normal distribution using the Lilliefors test (Norusis, 1993). The comparison of Lilliefors results for transformed and untransformed scales are presented in Table 4.3. Only the hypervigilance scale improved when a square root transformation was applied but even then it did not produce a satisfactory result when the Lilliefors test was applied. For all of the other scales no approximation of a normal distribution was obtained.

Factor analysis

All decision making items were submitted to factor analysis using orthogonal rotation and the number of factors was not specified. This approach was aimed at replicating the factor analysis conducted by Coulton and colleagues (1988).

Table 4.3
Lilliefors tests for normality for decision making scales, transformed and untransformed

Scale	Skew	Kurtosis	Statistic	Significance
Hypervigilance	.6641	-.1750	.0970	.0001
Square root hypervigilance	.3199	-.7145	.0086	.0008
Restricted choice	-.1528	-1.3001	.1092	.0000
Square root restricted choice	-.4394	-1.0583	.1213	.0000
Rushed	1.1527	.2243	.2811	.0000
Square root rushed	.8654	-.5543	.2975	.0000
Family support	-1.6582	2.2898	.2367	.0000
Control	-1.6404	2.1065	.2543	.0000
Certainty	-.9338	.4316	.1381	.0000

Table 4.4
Orthogonal factor analysis of decision
making variables (n = 194)

Variable	Factor					
	1	2	3	4	5	6
Hyper 1	.560	-.147	.131	-.368	-.056	.197
Hyper 2	.795	.192	-.010	-.040	-.017	-.089
Hyper 3	.643	.203	-.021	-.174	.065	-.229
Hyper 4	.162	.640	.082	-.222	-.158	.075
Hyper 5	.236	.444	-.335	-.015	.152	-.068
Hyper 6	.742	.190	-.055	-.080	.047	.043
Hyper 7	.284	.556	-.007	.203	.015	-.275
Family 1	.034	-.032	.023	.112	.860	.111
Family 2	-.238	.076	.035	-.047	.757	.284
Family 3	.225	-.148	.005	.079	.757	-.085
Restrict 1	.008	.009	.870	-.033	.036	-.097
Restrict 2	.032	-.029	.901	-.009	-.016	.019
Restrict 3	-.022	.253	.549	.127	.063	-.019
Certainty 1	-.100	-.064	.104	.699	.079	.139
Certainty 2	-.193	-.180	-.054	.712	.106	.087
Certainty 3	-.134	-.045	.004	.624	.037	.569
Certainty 4	-.031	-.026	.223	.394	-.154	.362
Control 1	-.062	-.128	-.076	.231	.106	.726
Control 2	-.069	.002	-.065	.045	.159	.772
Rushed 1	.077	.603	.073	-.446	-.022	-.012
Rushed 2	.051	.814	.157	-.059	-.054	-.055
Eigenvalue	4.13	2.19	2.16	1.62	1.34	1.21
Pct Variance	19.7	10.4	10.3	7.7	6.4	5.8

As expected, six factors were identified as outlined in Table 4.4. The correlation matrix for the decision making scales is presented in Table 4.5 (Appendix D).The requirement for the scales to be identified in a simple structure was only partially met. The indicators for the scales do not have high loadings on only one factor with low loadings on the other factors. The restricted choice scale and the family support scale were identified in a simple structure. However, factor four, the certainty scale, had one item which also loaded onto factor six, the control scale. This item is 'I had enough information about my condition to decide what to do' (certainty 3). In addition, some of the hypervigilance scale items, factor one, load onto factor two, the rushed scale. These items are 'I felt I had to decide quickly' (hypervigilance 4), 'I thought a great deal about what to do' (hypervigilance 5) and 'Everyone tried to tell me what to do' (hypervigilance 7). The latter item does not conceptually fit as it does not connote time pressure in decision making. Finally, the first item of the rushed scale, 'Everyone seemed quite rushed' also loaded onto the certainty scale factor. Given this result the construct validity of the rushed scale, which consists of only two items, must be questioned.

Internal consistency reliability

The six scales were subjected to internal consistency analysis using Cronbach's alpha. The results are shown in Table 4.6. The analysis indicated that reliability could not be improved by deletion of any items.

Table 4.6
Means, standard deviations (SD) and reliability coefficients (Alpha) of decision making scales (n = 194)

Scale	Number of items	Mean(SD)	Alpha
Hypervigilance	7	1.96 (.763)	.69
Family Support	3	4.29 (.993)	.73
Restricted Choice	3	3.19 (1.418)	.73
Certainty	4	4.06 (.858)	.69
Control	2	4.37 (.972)	.65
Rushed	2	1.93 (1.211)	.62

Disagreements

A substantial number of respondents indicated that they had disagreements about treatment or plans for the future while in the hospital as shown in Table 4.7. Almost half of the people interviewed indicated that there had been some disagreement during their hospital stay and the proportion of patients who reported having disagreements is similar for both social work and non social work patients. However, only 12 social work patients (13%) and 10 non social work patients (10%) indicated that the disagreements had made being in the hospital and planning for the future more difficult. Disagreements with family were less common with 20% of social work patients and 16% of non social work patients identifying that family disagreements occurred during their hospitalisation.

A number of people had disagreements in relation to more than one issue. The distribution of disagreements in relation to different issues is shown in Tables 4.8 and 4.9. In relation to disagreements with the hospital staff the reports by social work and non social work patients were surprisingly similar. More non social work patients commented on poor services provided by the hospital and about poor communication between themselves and doctors or nurses.

More social work patients reported disagreements in relation to their discharge destination (SW 11%, NSW 3%) and about the treatment planned for the post discharge period (SW 14%, NSW 10%).

Table 4.7
Frequency of disagreements between patients and hospital staff and between patients and family members (n = 194)

Disagreements	Hospital Staff n(%)	Family n(%)
No Disagreements	112 (57.7%)	159 (81.9%)
Disagreements	82 (42.3%)	35 (18.0%)
Total	194 (100%)	194 (100%)*

* Variation due to rounding

44

Table 4.8
Nature of disagreements with hospital staff for social work and non social work patients (n = 181)

Disagreement About	SW n(%)	NSW n(%)	Total n(%)
When discharged	20 (21%)	23 (26%)	43 (24%)
Treatment planned	21 (22%)	21 (24%)	42 (23%)
Services provided	13 (14%)	17 (19%)	30 (17%)
Treatment post discharge	13 (14%)	9 (10%)	22 (12%)
Treatment already given	11 (12%)	9 (10%)	20 (11%)
Where discharged to	10 (11%)	3 (3%)	13 (7%)
Poor communication	3 (3%)	5 (6%)	8 (4%)
Scheduling of treatment	2 (2%)	0 (0%)	2 (1%)
Access to medical record	1 (1%)	0 (0%)	1 (0%)
Total	94 (100%)	87(100%)	181 (100%)

In relation to family disagreements more social work patients reported having continuation of disputes that had commenced before their hospitalisation (SW 22%, NSW 12%). There were also more social work patients who reported family disagreement over treatment decisions (SW 22%, NSW 12%). These details about the nature of disagreements must be considered within the context of the small proportion of both groups of respondents who identified the disagreements as having a substantial impact on them and their well-being.

Outcome measures

Patient satisfaction with decisions

Patients were asked to rate on a six point scale ' How satisfied are you now with the decisions you made then (when in the hospital)'. The summary of responses is shown in Table 4.10. 78% of patients indicated that they were completely or very satisfied with the decisions made.

Table 4.9
Nature of disagreements with family for social work
and non social work patients (n = 61)

Disagreement About	SW n(%)	NSW n(%)	Total n(%)
Who would care for patient	7 (19%)	5 (20%)	12 (20%)
Treatment given to patient	8 (22%)	3 (12%)	11 (18%)
Continuation of previous disagreement	8 (22%)	3 (12%)	11 (18%)
Who managed home	3 (8%)	5 (20%)	8 (13%)
How home was managed	4 (11%)	2 (8%)	6 (10%)
Where discharged to	2 (5%)	2 (8%)	4 (6%)
Not specified	2 (5%)	1 (4%)	3 (5%)
Treatment planned	1 (3%)	0 (0%)	1 (2%)
Plans for future	0 (0%)	1 (4%)	1 (2%)
Financial issues	0 (0%)	1 (4%)	1 (2%)
Services at hospital	0 (0%)	1 (4%)	1 (2%)
When discharged	0 (0%)	1 (4%)	1 (2%)
Worry about patient's health	1 (3%)	0 (0%)	1 (2%)
Total	36 (100%)	25 (100%)	61 (100%)

Problems at time of interview and when in the hospital

Patients were asked a series of questions about problems they experienced at the time of the interview and when they were in the hospital. They were asked to identify whether they experienced problems in specific areas and to rate how serious those problems were.

In relation to problems experienced while they were in the hospital they were asked who helped them deal with the problems.

The types of problems most frequently experienced by patients are outlined in Tables 4.11 and 4.12. For both social work and non social work patients the most frequently occurring problems were the patient's adjustment to the illness, the family's adjustment to the illness, emotional problems, and financial problems. This was consistent for both time periods: that is, when the patient was in the hospital and after discharge. At the time of the interview patients reported few other problems than those presented to them. For social work patients the additional problems included the following:

- need for a machine to test a medical condition

- problems with the coordination of medical services

- cost of transport for frequent outpatient appointments

- other issues not specified.

For non social work patients the additional problems included:

- recuperating from surgery

- the effects of losing a child, and

- an unspecified legal/health problem.

In relation to problems experienced while in the hospital there were many more issues raised in addition to the list presented to respondents.

Table 4.10
Satisfaction with decisions for social work
and non social work patients (n = 193)

Level of Satisfaction	SW n(%)	NSW n(%)	Total n(%)
Not at all satisfied	3 (3%)	2 (2%)	5 (3%)
Not very satisfied	1 (1%)	0 (0%)	1 (0%)
Somewhat satisfied	6 (6%)	11 (11%)	17 (9%)
Quite satisfied	13 (14%)	6 (6%)	19 (10%)
Very satisfied	17 (18%	12 (12%)	29 (15%)
Completely satisfied	54 (57%)	68 (69%)	122 (63%)
Total	94(100%)*	99(100%)	193(100%)*

* Variation in total percentage due to rounding

Table 4.11
Distribution of types of problems experienced by social work and non social
work patients at time of interview (n = 192)

Type of Problem	SW(n = 94) n(%)	NSW(n = 98) n(%)	Total n(%)
Adjustment to illness	46 (49%)	32 (33%)	78 (41%)
Financial	36 (38%)	20 (20%)	56 (29%)
Emotional	24 (26%)	18 (18%)	42 (22%)
Family's adjustment to illness	27 (29%)	11 (11%)	38 (20%)
Work or school	21 (22%)	15 (15%)	36 (19%)
Family relationships	19 (20%)	6 (6%)	25 (13%)
Legal	14 (15%)	6 (6%)	20 (10%)
Accommodation	14 (15%)	3 (3%)	17 (9%)
Other relationships	9 (10%)	3 (3%)	12 (6%)
Other	6 (6%)	3 (3%)	9 (5%)

These included:

- complaints about lack of care from nursing staff (2 social work and 2 non social work patients),

- complaints about hospital services/discharge process (3 social work patients and 4 non social work patients),

- problems related to the patient's physical condition (2 social work patients and 2 non social work patients),

- problems with roommates in hospital (1 social work patient and 2 non social work patients),

- problems in relation to lack of access to family or providing care for family members (1 social work patient and 1 non social work patient),

- other individual issues such as problems with insurance companies and one patient complained about her doctor's personality.

Table 4.12
Distribution of types of problems experienced by social work and non social work patients when in the hospital (n = 192)

Type of Problem	SW(n = 94) n(%)	NSW(n = 98) n(%)	Total n(%)
Adjustment to illness	39 (41%)	28 (29%)	67 (35%)
Emotional	36 (38%)	20 (20%)	56 (29%)
Family's adjustment to illness	19 (20%)	15 (15%)	34 (18%)
Financial	17 (18%)	14 (14%)	31 (16%)
Work or school	10 (11%)	11 (11%)	21 (11%)
Family relationships	9 (10%)	8 (8%)	17 (9%)
Other relationships	8 (9%)	7 (7%)	15 (8%)
Accommodation	8 (9%)	3 (3%)	11 (6%)
Legal	7 (7%)	2 (2%)	9 (5%)
Other	12 (13%)	14 (14%)	26 (14%)

The patients also identified who helped them in relation to each individual problem they had while they were in the hospital. A summary of the people identified as helpers is presented in Table 4.13 (Appendix D). This was calculated by summing the total of responses for each helper over all problems. The social worker was included as an identified helper by 38 social work patients, which is 40% of the total group of social work patients. It is noticeable that the family was most frequently mentioned as providing assistance to patients.

While a number of patients stated that no one helped, there were a number of situations where they also specified that they did not ask for help or mention their problem to any hospital staff. For example, one patient did not have visits from his wife during his hospitalisation because they could not afford the fares for her to travel back and forth to the hospital. He was very distressed by this forced separation but he did not raise it as an issue because he had already obtained some assistance with medication expenses. In another instance a patient did not disclose to hospital staff the problems she was experiencing with her boyfriend. One young patient stated that the 'social worker did not have a chance because he didn't say a lot about his problems and he was in the hospital for such a short time'.

A wide variety of people were nominated as helpers in addition to hospital staff and family but they were not cited by more than a few patients. These other people nominated as helpers included friends, chaplains or ministers of religion, attorneys, other patients, students, work colleagues, physical therapists, counsellors from outside the hospital, a landlord, a rehabilitation conference, and prayer. Some patients identified themselves as the person who resolved the issue.

The differences between social work and non social work patients in terms of the problems experienced may also be examined by means of the total number of problems identified by patients. This is presented in Tables 4.14 and 4.15 (Appendix D). The social work patients appear to have had higher numbers of problems than the non social work patients both while in the hospital and after discharge.

The patient's ratings of problems were summed to form a 'problems now' and a 'problems then' score. In each case the highest possible problem score from ten items was 60. The distribution of problem scores is shown in Tables 4.16 and 4.17 (Appendix D). More non social work patients reported no problems both during their hospitalisation (SW 23, NSW 36) and after discharge (SW 23, NSW 45). In both groups there were few people recording scores above 30 either when in the hospital or at the time of the interview.

The intention was to use the 'problems then' and 'problems now' scores in the form of a post/then test in place of pre and post test scores. Since previous research has indicated that social work services are effective in reducing problems experienced by patients in the post discharge period (Oktay et al., 1992; Wolock, Schlesinger, Dinerman, and Seaton, 1987) the assumption was that, given the benefit of social work intervention, patients would experience fewer problems in the post discharge period.

The distribution of problem difference scores is shown in Table 4.18 (Appendix D). Positive scores indicate that a patient's situation had improved from the time when they were in the hospital. Negative scores indicate that the patient had higher levels of problem points at the time of the post discharge interview. A substantial number of patients, more than a third, had higher problem scores at the time of the interview than when in the hospital (SW 39, NSW 27, Total Group 35%). Approximately one third of patients showed no difference in the degree of problems experienced while they were in the hospital and afterwards (SW 21, NSW 38, Total Group 31%), and the final third seemed to have less difficulty after leaving hospital in comparison with when they were patients (SW 34, NSW 31, Total Group 35%) .

Tests of hypotheses

Facilitation of decision making and satisfaction with decisions made

The first hypothesis about the effects of the decision making environment in the hospital focused on whether patients who reported having positive support for decision making would also report a higher degree of satisfaction with those decisions.

Hypothesis 1: Patients who perceive their decision making as involving more family support, certainty about the future, and control over choices will have a higher level of satisfaction with decisions made in the hospital than those who perceive their decision making as involving less family support, less certainty about the future, and less control over decisions made.

Backward elimination regression analyses (Afifi and Clark, 1990) was used to test this hypothesis because use of this procedure examines the relationships between a number of independent variables in relation to the dependent variable, and allows the examination of the model which includes only those variables which contribute a significant amount of the explained variance to the dependent variable. All variables are entered in the first equation and in subsequent equations variables are eliminated one by one according to which variable accounts for the least variance in the dependent variable. The maximum probability of F-to-remove value was set at .10.

The initial equation submitted for analysis was:

$Y =$ $a + b_1$ control $+ b_2$ certainty $+ b_3$ family support $+ b_4$ age $+ b_5$ marital status $+ b_6$ gender $+ b_7$ ethnicity $+ b_8$ education $+ b_9$ gap between discharge and interview $+ b_{10}$ length of stay $+ b_{11}$ category as social work or non social work $+ e$.

In relation to this hypothesis the dependent variable satisfaction with decisions made while in the hospital included the three facilitator decision making scales of control, certainty, and family support as the independent variables. The control variables included are listed below:

- Patient's *age* which was recorded in years.

- Patient's *marital status* as a binary variable (0 not married, 1 married or with partners).

- Patient's *gender* was indicated by 0 for male and 1 for female.

- Patient's *ethnicity* was also coded in binary form (0 non white, 1 white). This variable was recoded from the original seven categories because of the predominance of white American patients in the sample.

- Patient's *education* which was recorded as years of education completed.

- The gap between discharge date and interview date was recorded in days. This variable was included because there was the possibility that the difference in timing of the interview may influence results.

- Patient's *length of stay* in the hospital was recorded in days.

- Patient's *category* was defined as social work patient, coded 1, or non social work patient, coded 0.

The variable of income level could not be included because of the high number of cases missing data for that variable. Analysis of the difference between social work and non social work patients was carried out by a procedure of repeating the regression equation for each sub group so that the results could be compared.

Table 4.19 presents the results of the backward elimination regression analysis. The correlation matrix, Table 4.20, is in Appendix D. In the final equation the control scale (b = .229, p < .01) and the certainty scale (b = .472, p < .001) demonstrated positive and significant relationships with satisfaction with decisions made. In addition, the patients' age (b = .010, p < .05) and being white rather than not white (b = .371, p < .05) were shown to be positively and significantly related to satisfaction ratings. The family support scale and control variables of marital status, gender, the gap between discharge and interview date and patients' length of stay in the hospital were all excluded from the final equation. The control variable of whether the patient was a social work patient or a non social work patient was also not shown to be significantly related to the satisfaction rating in this equation.

The R squared value shows that the variables included in this analysis account for only a moderate proportion of the variance in satisfaction ratings.

The control and certainty scales together, with the age and ethnicity variables, may be described as the most concise model for this set of independent variables in relation to satisfaction with decisions made. In these results there may be some influence from the moderate correlation between the control and certainty scales but the collinearity was not sufficient to cause removal of either variable from the equation.

Table 4.19

Backward elimination regression analysis of satisfaction with decisions on selected independent variables (n = 193)

Variables	b	SE	β	F
Control Scale	.229	.087	.182	6.849**
Certainty Scale	.472	.099	.331	22.887***
Age	.010	.005	.138	4.713*
Ethnicity[a]	.371	.182	.130	4.153*

R^2 = .249
Adjusted R^2 = .234

$* p < .05, ** p < .01, *** p < .001$

a.   Ethnicity in terms of white, coded 1, versus not white, coded 0.

Given the low R squared these results may be regarded as giving an indication of some variables which may contribute variation in satisfaction ratings for this group of patients. These findings indicate that the higher the scores on the control and certainty scales and the older the patient, the higher were their ratings of satisfaction with decisions made. There is also an indication that white patients were more likely to record higher satisfaction scores than non white patients. This analysis did not demonstrate any significant difference between the satisfaction ratings of social work and non social work patients.

To examine this more closely the same regression equation was submitted after splitting the file so that separate analysis for social work and non social work patients could be performed. The initial equation presented above was used for these analyses. This clarifies the relationships between the variables to some extent. The regression analysis for the non social work patients, shown in Table 4.21, reveals that for this group the certainty scale (b = .766, p < .001) and being white in comparison with being not white (b = .533, p < .05) are significantly related to satisfaction with decisions made. This indicates that for this group of non social work patients, those who were white and who scored higher on the certainty scale were likely to express higher satisfaction with the decision making while they were in the hospital. The correlation matrix is presented in Table 4.22 in Appendix D.

Table 4.21
Backward elimination regression analysis of satisfaction with decisions on selected independent variables: non social work patients (n = 99)

Variables	b	SE	β	F
Certainty Scale	.766	.118	.531	42.302***
Education	-.060	.033	-.144	3.186
Ethnicity[a]	.533	.233	.187	5.221*

R^2 = .387
Adjusted R^2 = .368

* p < .05, *** p < .001

a. Ethnicity in terms of white, coded 1, versus not white, coded 0.

For the social work group of patients the results are in Table 4.23. The certainty scale (b = .298, p < .05) and the patient's age (b = .015, p < .05) are shown to be positively and significantly related to satisfaction ratings. For this group of social work patients having higher certainty scores and being older were associated with higher ratings of satisfaction. The low R squared indicates that there are other factors not included in this equation which may influence the social work patients' level of satisfaction with decision making.

Taken together the separate analyses for social work and non social work patients indicate that there are differences between the two groups in the variables which might be said to influence satisfaction ratings. However, there is no indication that the two groups differ in terms of level of satisfaction reported. For both groups certainty about the outcomes, as measured by the certainty scale, is associated with higher levels of satisfaction. In each group one other factor demonstrates an influence on satisfaction ratings. For the social work group it is the patient's age and for the non social work group it is whether the patient was white or not.

Considering the problems with the decision making scales in relation to deviation from normal distribution, the lack of clear definition of the certainty and control scales from the factor analysis, and the modest reliability coefficients, there is need for caution in deriving any conclusions from these results.

Table 4.23
Backward elimination regression analysis of satisfaction with decisions on selected independent variables: social work patients (n = 94)

Variables	b	SE	β	F
Control Scale	.290	.149	.204	3.764
Certainty Scale	.298	.145	.212	4.211*
Age	.015	.007	.203	4.272*

$R^2 = .172$
Adjusted $R^2 = .144$

* $p < .05$

It is not possible to suggest either that there is support or lack of support for the hypothesis. All that may be stated is that there is an indication from these results that certainty about outcomes and the patient's perception of control over choices may have some association with the level of satisfaction with decisions made and that family support may not be a relevant variable to include in further studies. There is also the likelihood that other factors also influence level of satisfaction with decisions.

Facilitation of decision making and psychosocial outcomes

The second hypothesis was concerned with the impact of positive aspects of decision making on psychosocial outcomes.

Hypothesis 2: Family support, certainty about the future, and control over choices in decision making are positively associated with positive psychosocial outcomes.

Two measures of psychosocial outcomes have been used: *problem difference scores*, and *problems at the time of the interview*. The first measure, problem difference scores, was calculated by subtracting the problem score at the time of the interview from the problem score when the patient was in the hospital. This problem difference score was intended to reflect the change associated with social work intervention. As shown by the frequencies of scores it appears that the people who reduced their problem score were balanced by people who increased their problem score in the post hospital period. Because of this it was anticipated that regression analysis would not produce meaningful results and so the problems score at the time of the interview was added as an additional measure of pyschosocial outcome.

Using the Lilliefors statistic the problem difference score was shown to be significantly different from a normal distribution (Lilliefors .1210, p < .001) and none of the attempted transformations improved the result. The problems score at the time of the interview (Lilliefors .1703, p < .000) showed a similar significant deviation from normal distribution but this was remedied by a natural log transformation (Lilliefors .0696, p > .2000). Since different results were obtained when using the transformed dependent variable this was the one used for all analyses involving problems scores at the time of the interview.

The backward elimination regression equation with problem difference scores as the dependent variable and the same group of independent variables used for hypothesis one. The final equation identified family support (b = 1.086, p < .01) as the only independent variable positively and significantly related to the dependent variable as shown in Table 4.25. The correlation matrix, Table 4.26, is presented in Appendix D. The results indicate that there is no significant relationship between problem difference scores and the category as a social work or non social work patient.

Table 4.25
Backward elimination regression analysis of problem difference scores on selected independent variables (n = 190)

Variables	b	SE	β	F
Family Support Scale	1.086	.395	.195	7.546**
Gender	1.564	.828	.134	3.568

$R^2 = .058$
Adjusted $R^2 = .048$

** p < .01

This was opposite to the expected result. These results imply that the higher the family support score the higher the problem difference score. Given the extremely low R squared it might be suggested that the results may be disregarded as it may be hypothesised that other factors account for the variance in problem difference scores. However, no firm conclusions may be drawn from these results because of the inadequacies in the decision making scales as presented earlier.

Log of problems at time of interview

An additional analysis was undertaken using the log of problems at the time of the interview (problems now) as a psychosocial outcome variable. The independent variables included the same variables used in previous regression equations. The log transformation of problem now scores resulted in additional loss of cases and so the analysis was done using only 122 of the original sample. The results are shown in Table 4.27. Table 4.28 containing the correlation matrix is in Appendix D.

Only the family support scale (b = -.199, p < .05) and category as social work or non social patient (b = .553, p < .01) were identified as significantly related to the problem scores at the time of the interview. For this sample social work patients, in comparison with non social work patients, were likely to have higher problems score at the time of the interview. The relationship between family support and problems at the time of the interview was inverse indicating that the higher the perceived family support the lower the problems score. Because of the small sample size no split file analysis could be performed.

The low R squared might be taken as an indication that other factors in addition to family support and whether or not patients were seen by social workers affect the level of problems patients experience after discharge. The family support scale was clearly defined in the factor analysis and also demonstrated an acceptable reliability coefficient but the problems with the structure of the decision making scales overall, and the lack of approximation to normal distribution, make it difficult to be confident about the meaning to be attributed to these results.

As in relation to the first hypothesis there can be no firm conclusions reached about the influence of the decision making environment on psychosocial outcomes for this group of patients from the results of this study. It is reasonable to suggest that the link between family support and patients' experience of psychosocial problems after discharge is worthy of further examination.

Inhibitors to decision making and psychosocial outcomes

The third hypothesis is concerned with the effect of negative aspects of decision making on psychosocial outcomes.

Table 4.27

Backward elimination regression analysis of problems at time of interview scores on selected independent variables (n = 122)

Variables	b	SE	β	F
Certainty Scale	-.147	.083	-.153	3.154
Family Support Scale	-.199	.078	-.224	6.584*
Category: Social Work[a]	.522	.165	.298	9.998**
Gap: Discharge to Interview	.010	.005	.189	3.905

$R^2 = .149$
Adjusted $R^2 = .120$

* p < .05, ** p < .01

a. Social work category coded 1 for social work patients and 0 for non social work patients

Hypothesis 3: The association between the negative aspects of decision making (hypervigilance, disagreements, restricted choices and little time) and negative psychosocial outcomes for the patient decrease substantially for patients who received social work intervention. The assumption was that there would be a stronger inverse relationship between the inhibitor decision making scales and psychosocial outcomes for those patients who did not receive social work services.

The initial equation submitted for analysis was:

Y $= a + b_1$ hypervigilance $+ b_2$ restricted choice $+ b_3$ rushed $+ b_4$ number of disagreements with hospital staff $+ b_5$ number of disagreements with family $+ b_6$ age $+ b_7$ marital status $+ b_8$ gender $+ b_9$ ethnicity $+ b_{10}$ education $+ b_{11}$ gap between discharge and interview $+ b_{12}$ length of stay $+ b_{13}$ category as social work or non social work $+ e$.

As with the earlier hypothesis, hypothesis 2, separate analyses were completed using the dependent variables of problem difference scores and the problems scores at the time of the interview. The independent variables included the inhibitor decision making scales of *hypervigilance, restricted choice and time pressure*. The hypervigilance scale was transformed into square root hypervigilance in order to increase the approximation toward a normal distribution. However, after comparing results using the transformed and the original hypervigilance variable no significant differences were obtained. Therefore, in all regression equations the original hypervigilance variable was used.

Other variables included in the equations include those concerning disagreements between patients and hospital staff or between patients and family members. These variables were as follows:

- The *number of disagreements with hospital staff* defined in terms of the number of areas of the seven areas specified in the questionnaire (Appendix C). The seven areas were the kind of treatment planned, the treatment that had been given, the hospital services, when the patient would be discharged, where the patient would go after leaving hospital, treatment after leaving hospital and any other issues. Respondents identified disagreements in these area with yes/no responses.

- The *number of disagreements with family members* defined in terms of the number of areas of the seven areas specified in the questionnaire (Appendix C). The seven areas included disagreements about the treatment the patient was having, who would manage home and responsibilities while the patient was in the hospital, home and responsibilities not being looked after properly while the patient was in the hospital, who would look after the patient after discharge, where the patient would go after discharge, continuation of disagreements before hospitalisation and any other issues. Respondents identified disagreements in these area with yes/no responses.

The control variables included patient category, marital status, and gender as used in previous analyses. The regression was conducted using the backward elimination sequential procedure with listwise deletion of missing data.

The results of the equation with the problem difference scores as the dependent variable are shown in Table 4.29. The correlation matrix, Table 4.30, is presented in Appendix D.

No significant differences associated with whether patients were seen by a social worker were defined by this equation. The only variable shown to have a positive and significant relationship with problem difference scores was marital status (b = 1.608, p < .05). The implication of this result is that married people were likely to have higher problem difference scores that those who were not married in this group of patients.

With the regression analysis using log of problems at the time of the interview as the outcome variable the results are somewhat different as shown in Table 4.31.

Table 4.29
Backward elimination regression analysis of problem difference scores on selected independent variables (n = 190)

Variables	b	SE	β	F
Rushed	.638	.329	.138	3.752
Category: Social Work[a]	-1.418	.793	-.128	3.197
Marital Status[b]	1.608	.798	.143	4.060*
Gender	1.567	.827	.134	3.595

R^2 = .075
Adjusted R^2 = .055

* $p < .05$

a. Social work category coded 1 for social work patients and 0 for non social work patients
b. Marital Status coded 1 to indicate married and 0 to indicate not married.

The correlation matrix, Table 4.32, is in Appendix D. The hypervigilance scale (b = .310, $p < .01$), the rushed scale (b = -.161, $p < .05$), the number of disagreements with hospital staff (b = .112, $p < .05$), category as a social work or non social patient (b = .468, $p < .01$), and years of education (b = .050, $p < .05$), were all significantly related to the problems score at the time of interview. All of these apart from the rushed scale were positively related to the problems score.

These results imply that patients who were more anxious about decisions to be made while they were in the hospital, and who had higher numbers of disagreements with hospital staff at that time, also had more difficulties in the psychosocial problem areas discussed with them some time after discharge. The analysis indicates that this was more likely to be so for the more highly educated and for those who were social work patients.

The inverse relationship between being rushed and problem scores does not make sense theoretically as it suggests that patients who were less rushed when making decisions while they were in the hospital had a higher level of psychosocial difficulty in the post discharge period. This is opposite to what was hypothesised. The moderate correlation between the rushed scale and the hypervigilance scale and the lack of clear definition of the rushed scale as shown in the factor analysis results may have contributed to this result.

Table 4.31

Backward elimination regression analysis of problems at time of interview scores on selected independent variables (n = 122)

Variables	b	SE	β	F
Hypervigilance	.311	.113	.279	7.563**
Rushed	-.161	.068	-.229	5.588*
Number Disagreements: Hospital Staff	.112	.052	.193	4.601*
Number Disagreements: Family	.135	.077	.151	3.059
Category: Social Work[a]	.468	.161	.268	8.451**
Education	.049	.024	.166	4.076*
Marital Status[b]	-.281	.144	-.162	3.775
Gap: Discharge to Interview	.009	.005	.173	3.497

$R^2 = .259$
Adjusted $R^2 = .206$

* $p < .05$, ** $p < .01$

a. Social work category coded 1 for social work patients and 0 for non social work patients
b. Marital Status coded 1 to indicate married and 0 to indicate not married.

The modest R squared value indicates that other variables not included in this analysis have an influence on the degree of problems experienced by patients after discharge from hospital.

In relation to the decision making scales there can be little certainty about the meaning of the results obtained. The decision making environment may well have had some impact on the level of problems experienced by this group of patients after discharge. The results indicating a relationship between having a higher level of problems after discharge and the other variables might be considered to be more meaningful. However, the correlation matrix shows that the number of disagreements with hospital staff has a moderate correlation with the hypervigilance scale and this too may have had an impact on the results.

5 Results: Utilisation of social work resources

This chapter presents the findings in relation to the data on costs and use of social work time. After an outline of the descriptive statistics the findings from regression analyses to identify cost drivers are presented.

The final hypothesis was focused on exploration of factors associated with increased use of social work resources.

Hypothesis 4: The patient's experience of disagreements in decision making, the number and type of problems experienced by the patient, the patient's ethnicity, and length of stay in hospital are related to higher use of social work resources.

Measures of resource utilisation

The primary measure of social work resource for this study is *total case costs* defined as the cost of social work time, supervision time, training time, any other time, the supervisor's time, parking subsidy and any other expenses as identified by the social workers. The total case costs variable was not as comprehensive in coverage of cost factors as was intended and the number of patients for which there were costs in addition to social work time were few. Therefore, another dependent variable used was *cost of total social work time* which included the costs of social work time in service delivery, supervision time, training time, other time and the supervisor's time.

This was selected as being more meaningful in analysis of the cost drivers in relation to use of social work resources. The cost of total social work time includes more components of time than has been recorded in previous social work productivity studies (Coulton et al., 1985; Semke et al., 1993). It is also the more logical measure of resource utilisation when a full analysis of all costs, including fixed costs, cannot be calculated and when some categories of additional costs apply to only a few cases. Neither of these measures have been studied previously in relation to social work service delivery in hospitals.

Descriptive statistics

Social work time utilisation

The summary data of social work time expenditure per patient is provided in Table 5.1. This table includes a summary of social work service delivery time expenditure for the study admission (the admission that resulted in their selection into the study) and social work time expenditure for all other admissions during 1995 (the admissions which preceded the study admission during 1995). Supervision time, training time and other time is not included here.

Table 5.1
Distribution of social work service delivery time expenditure during study admission and during other admissions in 1995
(n = 94)

| Time (hours) | Admission | |
	Study n(%)	Other in 1995 n(%)
None	0 (0%)	64 (68%)
Under 1 hour	28 (30%)	6 (6%)
1 to 1.99	42 (45%)	6 (6%)
2 to 2.99	13 (14%)	6 (6%)
3 to 4.99	6 (6%)	5 (5%)
5 to 7.9	2 (2%)	1 (1%)
8 to 10.99	3 (3%)	5 (5%)
20 to 20.99	0 (0%)	1 (1%)
Mean (SD): 1.905 (1.836)		
Total	94 (100%)	94 (100%)*

* Variation in total percentage due to rounding.

64

For approximately two thirds of the social work patients the study admission was their only admission for 1995. Most often the social work patients in this group received very brief intervention. Three quarters of these patients received social work intervention amounting to two hours or less, and more than 80% of them received 3 hours or less. Fewer than 5 patients received 10 hours or more of social work resource time overall.

Most of the social work time was spent in activities related to direct service delivery to patients and most social workers did not require supervision or consultation in relation to these patients. Eighteen social workers reported supervision time in relation to the study patient and in most instances it was estimated that only 5 minutes was spent in discussing the patient (for 8 patients). In 3 cases supervision time was recorded as half an hour, and for one case 2 hours of supervision or consultation were required.

The patients described the social work intervention time as even more brief than the time allocations recorded by social workers. This is not surprising as social workers do part of their work in the office when contacting other agencies or when interviewing family members so that not all social work intervention is conducted in face to face contact with the patient. From the patients' viewpoint the mean social work contact time was approximately 15 minutes (SD = .568 hours). However, only 37 patients were able to estimate how much time the social worker had spent with them.

The social workers recorded very little time devoted to reading, study or training that was directly related to work with individual patients. Only 3 social workers identified training time related to the study patient and the time expenditure in training was small, amounting to 20 minutes or less. Only five social workers reported other time and each one specified one hour of other activities (e.g. making telephone calls from home, attending a meeting in another agency related to the patient's care, education session for hospital staff about the patient).

Costs

As might be expected the low time per patient translates into low costs per patient in terms of the calculations for this study. The details are provided in Table 5.2. The lowest total case cost for a social work service to this sample of patients was $4.75 and the highest was $385.79. The highest total social work time cost (service delivery time, supervision time, training time and other time) was $239.45. For more than three quarters of this sample social work intervention cost $50.00 or less. There is no published material providing statements of expected costs per case for hospital social work but given estimates of $6,462 as an average hospital charge (Saffran and Phillips, 1989) and $900.00 per bed day for nursing facilities (Concannon, 1995), the maximum cost of $239.00 for social work services in an acute care teaching hospital appears modest.

Table 5.2

Distribution of costs of total social work time expenditure
and total costs (n = 94)

| Time (dollars) | Total Costs | |
	Social Work Time n(%)	Case Costs n(%)
No cost[a]	8 (0%)	8 (0%)
Up to $10.00	5 (0%)	5 (0%)
$10.01 to $20.00	15 (16%)	14 (15%)
$20.01 to $30.00	22 (23%)	21 (22%)
$30.01 to $40.00	14 (15%)	13 (14%)
$40.01 to $50.00	9 (10%)	10 (11%)
$50.01 to $100.00	14 (15%)	12 (13%)
$100.01 to $200.00	6 (6%)	6 (6%)
$200.01 to $400.00	1 (1%)	5 (5%)
Mean (SD):	40.31 (42.13)	49.97 (64.22)
Total	94 (100%)*	94 (100%)*

* Variation in total percentage due to rounding

a. Some intern cases where the intern required no supervision time result in no cost
to the social work department when costs are calculated on a case product basis.

Parking subsidies were provided for only 5 patients in the sample. The value of
the parking assistance was considerable when it was provided. The least expensive
parking assistance provided was to the value of $56.00 and the highest amounted
to $351.00. Only one social worker identified other costs of $25.00.

Testing of hypotheses

The regression analyses were aimed at identification of cost drivers for utilisation
of social work resources by this sample of patients in this particular hospital. Two
sets of analyses were conducted with dependent variables of total case cost and
total social work time cost.

Stepwise regression analysis with listwise deletion of missing data was used so that the contribution of the different independent variables might be examined. Stepwise regression analysis is a sequential entry procedure which combines the approaches of forward and backward elimination procedures (Afifi and Clark, 1990). As with forward stepwise selection the first variable selected is that with the largest correlation with the dependent variable. Subsequent variables are added depending on the magnitude of the partial correlations. The stepwise procedure repeats the calculations with different sub sets of the total pool of independent variables, defining which variables are included or excluded based on the significance level obtained for each variable. The procedure involves computation of the equations on the basis of probability of F-to-enter and probability of F-to-remove values. The process stops when no variables can be added or removed based on the F values. This approach to analysis provides for examination of different clusters of variables and provides information about the contribution of each variable to the explained variance. The probability F-to-enter value used was .05 and the probability F-to-remove was .10 for these analyses.

In this context there is a need for stepwise regression methods. There is not a well developed theory about what constitutes the significant set of cost drivers for social work activity in hospital settings. There are some indications from previous research and this study attempts to add to what has been identified to date.

For these analyses intern cases which incurred no cost were removed from the sample. This resulted in a reduction of the sample size to eighty-six.

Independent variables

The independent variables included the following:

- *Patient disagreements with hospital staff.* This consisted of 7 binary variables coded 0 for no disagreement and 1 for disagreement. The areas were disagreements about treatment planned, about treatment already given, about hospital services, about when the patient would be discharged, about to where the patient would be discharged, about treatment post hospital, and any other disagreements. The two variables related to discharge planning were selected for inclusion because among the issues explored with patients discharge planning is the one most directly linked to social work activity (Dobrof, 1991; Kadushin and Kulys, 1993).

- *Patient disagreements with family members.* As in relation to disagreements with hospital staff these variables were in binary form. The areas included disagreement about treatment the patient was having, about who would manage the patient's home while the patient was in hospital, about how the patient's home was managed, about who cares for the patient at home, about to where the patient would be discharged, about other issues that were a

67

continuation of previous disagreements in the family and any other disagreements. Once again the two items concerned with discharge planning were included in the regression equation.

- The *number of problems* experienced by the patient while in hospital. This was measured by summing the number of problems the patient indicated were relevant from the list of ten presented to them as described above.

- The patient's *ethnicity*, a binary variable coded 0 for not white and 1 for white.

- The patient's *length of stay* in hospital recorded in days.

- The patient's *income* coded as an ordinal variable (Appendix C) but treated as if it were an interval scale.

Disagreements with hospital staff and resource utilisation

The first regression analyses were in relation to the disagreements with hospital staff together with variables used in previous studies including length of stay, number of problems, ethnicity and income.

The results of the stepwise regression equation with the dependent variable total case costs are presented in Table 5.3. The correlation matrix, Table 5.4, is in Appendix D. The results show none of the disagreement variables significantly related to total case costs. The length of stay variable (b = 2.853, p < .01) is the only variable retained in the equation but the R squared is very small. Length of stay is identified as significantly and positively related to total case costs. This is consistent with previous findings (Coulton et al., 1985; Semke et al., 1993) which indicate that the longer patients stay in hospital the more social work resources they utilise.

When the analysis was conducted using costs of total social work time as the dependent variable both family disagreements about to where the patient would be discharged (b = 81.731, p < .01) and income (b = -6.321, p < .05) were added to length of stay (b = 2.932, p < .001) as variables significantly related to costs as shown in Table 5.5. The correlation matrix, Table 5.6, is in Appendix D. These results imply that patients in lower income brackets who have longer stays in hospital receive more attention from social workers and this is what would be expected given the social work focus on vulnerable and disadvantaged populations. The disagreement variable indicates that where there is family disagreement about where the patient will go after leaving the hospital there is likely to be more use of social work time.

The other disagreement variables and the number of problems variable showed no significant relationship with social work time costs. The lack of relationship

68

Table 5.3
Stepwise regression analysis of total case costs on selected independent variables (n = 77)

Variables	Variables in the equation			Variables not in the equation	
	b(SE)	Beta	t value	Partial Corr.	t value
Length of stay	2.853(1.058)**	.297	2.697		
Hospital disagreement:					
When discharged				.222	1.965
Where discharged				.016	.141
Family disagreement:					
Who cares for				.204	1.800
Where discharged				.160	1.390
Number of problems				.136	1.179
Income				-.172	- 1.507
Ethnicity				-.006	- .055

R² = .088
Adjusted R² = .076

** p < .01

between number of problems and resource utilisation is opposite to the findings from other studies. In previous studies the number of problems was significantly related to social work time expenditure. In one study (Coulton et al., 1985) the number of problems addressed by the social worker was the strongest predictor of time expenditure when length of stay was not included in the equation. In the other study which used stepwise regression analysis (Semke et al., 1993) the number of assessed problems was one of the variables included in the model with best explanatory power. In both of these studies the number of problems were defined by the social workers and not by the patients and this difference may contribute to the variation in findings.

Types of problems and resource utilisation

An aim of this study was to explore whether it was possible to identify which kinds of problems experienced by patients were associated with higher utilisation of social work resources. Stepwise regression equations were conducted using both total case costs and total social work time costs as dependent variables. The independent variables were the items where patients rated themselves on a six point scale of degree of seriousness of problems experienced while they were in the hospital. Patients were asked to identify if they had problems in the specified areas of accommodation, finances, adjustment to illness, family's adjustment to illness, family relationships, other relationships, emotional issues, work or school, legal or other problems while they were in the hospital.

The regression analysis using total case costs as the dependent variable resulted in none of the variables being retained in the equation. When total social work time costs was used as the dependent variable only the variable problems at work or school (b = 6.944, p < .05) was shown as significant. These results are in Table 5.7 and the correlation matrix, Table 5.8, is in Appendix D. The types of problems variables show a number of moderate correlations which may have had an impact on the results and so little meaning can be derived from this finding.

These results suggest that when costs are measured in relation to social work time the patient's income level, the existence of family disagreement, and length of stay constitute the cost drivers for this particular group of patients. When type of psychosocial problems were considered only the problems about work or school were identified as a cost driver.

These results rely on acceptance of the data as accurate recordings of time expenditure, costs, and patient characteristics. The list of variables considered here is not exhaustive and the modest R squared indicates that there are other factors which influence resource utilisation in relation to social work services.

These findings together with the results in relation to the decision making scales are reviewed in the next chapter. At that point the implications of the findings are also considered.

Table 5.5

Stepwise regression analysis of total social work time costs on selected independent variables (n = 77)

Variables	Variables in the equation			Variables not in the equation	
	b(SE)	Beta	t value	Partial Corr.	t value
Length of stay	2.932(.577)***	.480	5.082		
Family disagreement:					
Where discharged	81.731(25.814)**	.299	3.166		
Income	-6.322(2.964)*	-.201	-2.133		
Hospital disagreement:					
When discharged				.171	1.475
Where discharged				.087	.738
Family disagreement:					
Who cares for				.033	.280
Number of problems				.195	1.684
Ethnicity				.097	.834

$R^2 = .363$
Adjusted $R^2 = .337$

* p < .05, ** p < .001, *** p < .001

Table 5.7

Stepwise regression analysis of total social work time costs on selected independent variables: types of problems

(n = 86)

Problems	Variables in the equation			Variables not in the equation	
	b(SE)	Beta	t value	Partial Corr.	t value
Work or school	6.944(3.108)*	.237	2.234		
Accommodation				-.156	-1.444
Financial				.065	.591
Adjustment illness				.081	.741
Family adjustment				.029	.265
Family relationships				.032	.296
Other relationships				-.032	-.293
Emotional				.138	1.271
Legal				.103	.945
Other				-.077	-.701

$R^2 = .056$

Adjusted $R^2 = .045$

* $p < .05$

6 Discussion and implications

This chapter begins with a review of the study and then the findings presented earlier are discussed. In the final part of the chapter the implications of results are considered in relation to social work practice, social work management and research.

Review of the study

For this study subjects were randomly selected from the separate groups of social work patients and non social work patients. The patients in the non social work group were not matched to those in the social work group so that the differences between the two populations could be studied in the process of testing the study hypotheses. The bivariate analyses of the sample drawn from the hospital population have shown that there were no significant differences between the interviewed and non interviewed groups in gender or marital status. While there were significant differences in terms of geographical location or medical condition treated at hospital, the PRE measures produced low coefficients and it is reasonable to propose that the influence of the differences between the interviewed and non interviewed group on the results would not be very strong.

Although the social work and non social work samples were very similar there were some noticeable characteristics of this study population overall which must be considered in reviewing the findings. As a group of patients the people studied were predominantly white Americans of European origin which is the same as the composition of the hospital for the year of the study. In the inner city neighborhoods from which patients come to this particular hospital there is a large Hispanic, non English speaking population. Because of the language barrier this group was not adequately sampled. However, in relation to African Americans and Asians the study sample accurately reflected the hospital population. There were few Asians in the sample.

There was a loss of two thirds of respondents from the original pool of potential respondents. About 18% of those who received letters but who were not able to be interviewed should not have been included in the sample because they were not able to communicate because of language or physical barriers or because they had no telephone. Even with this adjustment only half of those contacted were interviewed. The group studied did not include those too ill to talk over the telephone (52), those who had moved from their original address or who were still in rehabilitation centers (66) as well as those who object to surveys or who had some other reason not specified (182). These are the people not represented and the potential influence of the missing group on the findings cannot be known. This compromises the selection process. Given that the purpose of random sampling procedures is to obtain a sample which represents the population in order to allow generalisations to be made, the loss of large numbers decreases the extent to which the group actually studied might be said to be representative of the whole.

The gap between date of discharge and time of interview varied for the different patients more than was planned and it was evident that there was, in general, a longer gap for non social work patients than for social work patients. Some patients were not interviewed for more than 2 months after discharge. This raises questions about the accuracy of memory although other researchers consider that a three month gap is acceptable (Cleary et al, 1991). Regardless of this, there is the possibility that this time difference might have influenced the nature of responses, and so the variable recording the time difference was included in most of the analyses.

There was also a difference between the sub groups, social work and non social work, in terms of the medical unit under which they were admitted to the hospital and this may have had an impact on findings. This was not explored through the regression analyses. The patients in this study were not evenly distributed between the different medical units and for a large number of medical unit categories there were very small numbers. Inclusion of these variables in the regression equations did not have the potential to give meaningful results.

This study has been an exploratory one and much of the survey instrument was developed specifically for this study. There was no check to assess to what extent patients were giving socially desirable responses (De Vellis, 1991) as there was not sufficient space to incorporate this kind of measure in a thirty minute telephone interview. The decision making scales, which had been validated previously by Coulton and colleagues (1988) using confirmatory factor analysis, showed acceptable but not high alpha levels when submitted for internal consistency analysis in the current study. In addition the factor analysis did not reproduce exactly the distribution of items to the identified factors representing aspects of the decision making environment. In particular the rushed scale does not have a sufficient number of items with a coherent conceptual structure to warrant confidence in its use. Finally, many of the variables did not demonstrate a normal distribution and few were able to be successfully transformed to approximate normal distribution.

The attempt to produce a substitute pre/post test through use of post/then questioning did not succeed. The problem difference score, the difference between problem scores when in the hospital less the problem score at the time of the interview, produced results which showed that about the same number of people had a worsened situation after discharge as the number whose situation had improved. This result may represent more a limitation in relation to the theoretical model rather than inadequacy of the post/then procedure or the structure of the problem difference score. That is, the findings may be because it is not reasonable to expect that brief social work intervention will have a significant impact on the lives of seriously ill patients who face a number of health related as well as psychosocial problems.

Because of the unexpected results in relation to the problem difference scores, the problems score at the time of the interview was used as an outcome measure on its own. There must be questions about the adequacy of this score as an outcome measure for social work intervention.

There were limitations to other parts of the instrument. In this study there was no attempt to define or describe the nature of social work intervention while there was an attempt to measure outcomes. The importance of defining the nature of the intervention is understood (Reid, 1987) but it would need to be done in another study devoted exclusively to measurement of outcomes. The single question measure of satisfaction with decisions made while in hospital is acknowledged as inadequate but it was the only possible measure in the context of a telephone interview.

For the costing process the major deficiency of the study is that the data of social work time input was collected retrospectively from records and from social workers' reports some time after the social work intervention had been completed. There may have been a variety of motivations influencing how social workers recorded the time spent with patients (Grasso and Epstein, 1988) and there may well have been systematic variation in the way individual social workers calculated their time input. Given the pressure of work tasks for this group of workers it is unlikely that they would have been prepared to provide careful records of time utilisation specifically for this study and so the available data was the best that could be obtained at the time. The bias from retrospective data may only be surmised and it has to be hoped that the errors were randomly distributed.

The data about costs per worker were accurate in relation to the salary scale in operation at the time of the study and the details of parking and other expenses must be accepted as likely to be accurate. It would have been surprising if the hospital had been prepared to give full details of the social work department budget to an independent researcher and so the lack of complete costing information is understandable.

Given all these factors and the relatively modest sample size of 94 social work patients and 100 non social work patients there are severe constraints on what might be concluded from the data analysis. The findings here can only be taken to apply to this particular group of hospital patients and must be considered in the context of the deficiencies with the instruments used. This specification applies throughout this analysis of the results.

Decision making

Satisfaction with decisions made while in hospital

In relation to the first hypothesis about the influence of facilitator decision making aspects on level of satisfaction with decisions made, the finding of note is that family support and satisfaction with decisions are not related. The control and certainty scales, together with the age variable, were positively related to level of satisfaction when the results for the total sample were analysed. Non social work patients who were white were more likely to present higher satisfaction scores and for that group certainty about outcomes rather than control or family support was the variable which demonstrated significant association with satisfaction with decisions. For the group of social work patients more certainty about outcomes and being older were the factors associated with higher levels of satisfaction. The influence of ethnicity and age on reported satisfaction is consistent with the findings of a national study on patient satisfaction (Cleary et al., 1991). The interesting result from the current study is that the influence of ethnicity was not found for the social work patient group.

It is reasonable to accept that family support is not a significant factor in terms of satisfactions with decisions made. The patient may rightly perceive that the medical decision is one made by the patient and doctor and not by the family. The findings about control over choices and its relationship to satisfaction with decision making fits in with the literature which conveys that control over decision making is important for patients (Abramson, 1990; Coulton et al., 1989: Proctor et al.., 1993). This group of patients seemed to be well satisfied with their level of control over decisions. When asked at the end of the interview if they had as much control as they wanted over treatment and discharge decisions 89% answered affirmatively (SWP 87%, NSWP 90%). This was also reflected in the control scores where more than half of the patients interviewed recorded the highest possible control score (SWP 62%, NSWP 57%). The ratings of satisfaction with decision making were also skewed with most patients reporting a high level of satisfaction. This rating may have been influenced by their perceptions of health outcomes as patients who have good recovery from medical problems may be more likely to feel that they have made the right decisions as indicated by an earlier national patient satisfaction study (Cleary et al., 1991). However, as indicated by the recent RAND study (Marshall et al., 1996), the nature of the relationships between satisfaction with care and the patient's physical and mental heath status is not clear.

Another possibility is that the rating of satisfaction with decisions may be a result of cognitive dissonance in that the patients may 'enhance their opinions of decisions after they have made them' (Rosenfield, Kennedy, and Giacalone, 1987, p. 663). Nonetheless, the result indicates that patients who scored highly on the control scale were also likely to rate themselves highly satisfied with the decisions they made.

The relationship between certainty about outcomes and satisfaction indicates that patients who reported feeling certain about the outcomes while they were in the hospital were more likely to give high satisfaction scores at the time of the interview. This makes sense in that confidence that the doctors knew what they were doing, and a feeling that treatment results were predictable would be consistent with a sense of making the right decision in complying with treatment.

Facilitation of decision making and psychosocial outcomes

The second hypothesis sought to determine an association between the facilitator decision making scales and psychosocial outcomes. Two different outcome measures were used, problem difference scores, and problem scores at the time of the interview. The reason for this is that it was expected that social work patients would produce higher problem difference scores than non social work patients and lower problem scores at the time of the interview. In fact more social work patients reported problems both when in the hospital as well as at the time of interview in comparison with non social work patients. Also the ratings of severity of problems did not decline in the post discharge period. The consequent difficulties with the problem difference scores have already been described.

When the problem scores at the time of the interview were used as the dependent variable in the equation the variables that were significantly and positively related to problem scores were patient category as social work patient or non social work patient and family support. Social work patients were identified as having higher problem scores at the time of the interview when compared with non social work patients.

These results lead to a possible conclusion that social work patients are likely to have a higher degree of difficulty post discharge than those patients not seen by social workers while in the hospital and that the level of perceived family support rather than social work intervention is associated with positive outcomes.

The assumptions were that patients would have more problems while in the hospital than when at home and that social work intervention during hospitalisation would have an impact on those problems. The results do not support this hypothesis. There are good reasons why this may have occurred.

Firstly, there was generally a longer gap between discharge from hospital and interview for non social work patients (Table 4.11), with 43 social work patients interviewed within the first month after discharge and only 3 non social work patients interviewed in that time frame. There were twice as many non social work (81) as social work (40) patients interviewed between one and two months after discharge. This time factor may have influenced responses at the time of the interview especially in relation to memories of the time in hospital. However, the influence of this factor was incorporated into the regression equations through inclusion of the variable gap between interview and discharge. This variable did not show any significant relationship to the dependent variables in any of the equations. Bivariate analysis also showed no significant correlations between gap and any of the problem variables.

Another element to consider is the overall response of patients in identifying problems experienced when in the hospital and afterwards. Examination of the frequencies of problems at time of being in the hospital (Table 4.12) and at the time of the interview (Table 4.11) show that there was an increase in the frequency of problems for both groups of patients in a number of areas. The increases in problems after being discharged were in the areas of adjustment to illness, family adjustment to the patient's illness, financial issues, and problems at work or school. That is, there were more people reporting these problems at the time of the interview (Table 4.11) than when they reflected back to the time when they were in hospital (Table 4.12). This was so for both social work and non social work patients. In addition, in the social work group, but not in the non social work group, there was an increase in the number who reported problems with accommodation (while in hospital 8, at time of interview 14) and in family relationships (while in hospital 9, at time of interview 19) in the post discharge period.

The majority of these patients were in the hospital for a brief time and they were very ill while there. It is not surprising that adjustment to the illness for both patient and family might be important after discharge. Considering the context of hospital admission and treatment the increase in financial problems and work problems once at home is also to be expected. The difference between the social work and non social work groups in the areas of accommodation and family relationships is less easily explained.

These findings support the conclusions from earlier research that patients often need services post hospital regardless of whether or not they received social work services while in the hospital (Oktay et al., 1992). One group of researchers (Simon, Showers, Blumenfield, Holden, and Xiaochu, 1995) found that the week following discharge was the hardest for patients. This was not supported in this study which indicates that patients' problems persisted during the post hospital period and were not confined to the first week after discharge. Simon and colleagues (1995) were asking patients about post hospital services rather than about psychosocial problems. It is possible that patients may have a higher need for home nursing, home help and other services immediately after discharge. However, their problems in relation to the broad areas of psychological and social functioning which were discussed in this study may become more pressing after the initial recovery period has passed.

While the results in the current study confirm the importance of family support (Bergman et al, 1993; Wolock et al., 1987) as perceived by patients, there is no confirmation of the effectiveness of social work services in relation to problem reduction found by Oktay and others (1992).

In the social work literature there is a consistent theme about the importance of control over decision making (Abramson, 1990; Blazyk and Canavan, 1985; Blumenfield and Lowe, 1987; Brown and Furstenberg, 1992; Proctor et al., 1993). There is also an indication that from the patient's perspective this is not an absolute requirement, but one which varies according to individual characteristics and beliefs about locus of control (Coulton et al, 1989; Rotter, 1966). From the results in this study there is support for the importance of control as a factor which may be associated with the level of satisfaction but the issue of whether the patient felt they had control or not appears to have no relationship to the outcomes of intervention as measured by problem difference scores or the number of problems experienced after discharge.

Inhibitors to decision making and psychosocial outcomes

When the inhibitor decision making scales, hypervigilance, restricted choice and rushed, were entered into the equation together with the disagreements variables, it was expected that these negative factors would be negatively related to problem difference scores. That is, where there were inhibitors to decision making it was expected that patients would have more problems and that they would last longer. The results partially supported the hypothesis when the problems at the time of the interview was used as the outcome measure.

With the log of problems at the time of the interview as the dependent variable the hypervigilance scale, the number of disagreements with hospital staff, and patient category were all positively related to the problems score.

From these results, which are consistent with results in relation to the facilitator decision making scales, it is reasonable to suggest that where patients had anxiety about decisions while in the hospital and higher numbers of disagreements with hospital staff they had more problems after discharge. Of course this does not demonstrate a causal relationship and the problems with the decision making scales may negate these findings. However, it is possible that people with severe problems that persist over time (that is, before hospitalisation, during hospitalisation and after hospitalisation) may be the same people who experienced more stress in the decision making process and had problems in relationships with at least some hospital staff. The significance of the patient category variable indicates that social work patients, in comparison with non social work patients, have higher levels of problems in the post discharge period and this is consistent with the findings in relation to facilitator decision making scales.

Disagreements

Abramson and colleagues' (Abramson et al., 1993) analysis of two studies on disagreements in discharge planning found that social workers' perceptions were that 'disagreements occurred in at least one third of the cases, with most disagreements involving family members' (Abramson et al., 1993, p. 57). The information from the current study presents a different perspective in that it consists of the assessments made by patients rather than social workers. The study also includes disagreements of all types and not just those related to discharge planning. Overall, approximately 42% of patients in this sample reported disagreements with hospital staff and this applied to both social work (43.6%) and non social work patients (41%) (Table 4.7).

In one study reviewed by Abramson and colleagues there were more disagreements identified between patients and family members than between patients and social workers. In another study from the same review, patients were reported to have disagreements with hospital staff in 20% of the sample of cases and disagreements within the family were reported as occurring in approximately 18% of cases. The current study from the patients' perspective indicates that there were fewer disagreements between patients and family members (SWP 20%, NSWP 16%) than with hospital staff. However, the proportion of cases identified as involving family disagreement from social work and patient perspectives appears similar.

In the current study the disagreements with hospital staff were about treatment decisions as well as about discharge arrangements, with a higher incidence of disagreements about when the patient would be discharged than to where the patient would be discharged from hospital. In relation to disagreements with family members, the social work patients reported more ongoing family disagreements, disputes about treatment that had been given, and about who would care for the patient, than any other issues. For non social work patients the most frequently mentioned areas were in relation to who would care for the patient and who would manage the patient's home during the hospitalisation period.

While these results indicate a higher level of disagreements experienced by patients than has been described by social workers in previous studies, it must be considered in the context of the final question put to the respondents in this study. All patients were asked whether the disagreements that had occurred made being in the hospital and planning for the future more difficult for them. The predominant response was that the disagreements had been minor and with no long lasting effects. Only 22 of the 194 (SWP 12 or 13%, NSWP 10 or 10%) patients said that the disagreements that had occurred made being in the hospital and planning for the future more difficult for them.

Utilisation of social work resources

The second part of the study was focused on examination of the utilisation of social work resources by the 94 social work patients in this study. The intention was to identify factors, or cost drivers, which influence the use of social work resources. Because some interns did not receive supervision in relation to the work with the study patient the result was that their work with these patients resulted in no cost and so they were deleted from the sample. The regression analysis in relation to costs were conducted with data for 86 cases.

The pattern of resource utilisation

Previous studies of social work resource utilisation have identified patient's length of stay and the number of problems experienced by the patients as factors associated with use of social work time (Coulton et al., 1985; Semke et al., 1993; Spano and Lund, 1986). In each of these studies the dependent variable has been social work time per patient. Social work time was measured as time spent working with and on behalf of the patient.

Resource utilisation measured in terms of costs

For this study the resource utilisation has been defined in terms of costs. Two separate definitions of costs have been developed because the attempt to obtain total case costs was not successful. The costs additional to social work time costs that were obtained applied only to a few cases. Total case costs variable included all costs that could be identified as attributable to the services per patient. The total social work time costs incorporated all the costs for the social worker service delivery, training time, and the social work supervision for the services per patient. These definitions may be described as product costs based on variable costs which may be attributed to the product of the patient case. Fixed costs related to the operations of the social work department have not been allocated.

With total case costs there was an attempt to find all costs that could be attributed to the patients of social work services. The information provided indicated that costs for space, utilities, administrative support and consumables could not be allocated to individual staff or patients and so this costing has relied on the factors more obviously and clearly patient related. Whether because of inaccuracies in reporting, difficulty in remembering, or because it is the way things happened in fact, there were few cases where there were additional costs added to the labour based salary costs associated with service delivery, supervision and training. While there are inadequacies with these cost definitions they are more detailed than previous studies of hospital social work costs.

Unlike previous studies of the cost of social work services (Spano and Lund, 1986: Volland, 1980) the definitions of cost used in this study accounted for the different costs of social workers. The standard cost procedure used previously treats all social workers as if they are paid at the same rate when there is a substantial difference in salary between new graduates and senior practitioners. The attempt to incorporate non salary costs and to attribute those patient by patient where feasible has not resulted in improved understanding of costs in this situation. It is possible that there are other costs which might be attributed to patient care which have not been included in the total costs calculations. For example, there may be particular services supplied by the receptionist or administrative officers within the social work department that apply more to some groups of patients than to others.

The performance pressure on social workers

The changes in the health system over the past ten years are conveyed by the descriptive statistics from other studies in comparison with those from this study. In an earlier study (Coulton et al., 1985) the mean length of stay of patients for the study was 20.27 days (compared with a mean of 8.7 days for the hospital as a whole) whereas for this study the mean was 8.25 days (SD 7.166, median 6, mode 4) with the mean for the hospital only 5.49 days at the time of the study (Neeson, 1995). Parallel to this, the mean social work time expenditure for the 1985 study was 4.48 hours and for the current study the mean was 1.9 hours. In another study (Semke et al., 1993) the mean time expenditure was 3.87 hours.

These figures convey the pressure there has been to reduce length of stay in hospital and the impact of shorter length of stay for patients on social work services (Berger et al., 1996). Most importantly, it illustrates the difference in the way social workers were working in the different hospitals and time periods. The social workers in this study were allocating very small units of time to at least a proportion of the patients they served given that the mean time devoted to patients was less than two hours. Essentially, this means that in at least some cases social workers had little opportunity to assess what patients and families needed and then to provide the services required. With low investment of social work time per patient it is understandable that in this study the social work service delivery seems to be a very low cost enterprise with a mean total social work time cost of $40.31 per patient and the most expensive patient costing only $239.45.

The search for cost drivers

The hypothesis in relation to utilisation of social work resources was concerned with the search for the factors which influence how social work resources are used. What was being sought was information about the factors that might be identified as cost drivers for social work service delivery. The focus of this study was to identify as much as possible of the individual elements of social work time and other expenditures which could be attributed to the services required by the patient.

In this way the approach was similar to an activity based costing analysis at the product level of analysis. The product here was defined as the social work services to each individual patient. The search for cost drivers was done by conducting a series of stepwise regression equations.

A summary of the findings is presented in Table 6.1. This table shows the comparison of findings when the different dependent variables of *total case costs* and *total social work time costs* were used.

Regardless of the dependent variable in the equation there is a consistent finding that length of stay is significantly and positively related with use of resources.

This finding repeats the results from the previous studies (Coulton et al., 1985; Semke et al, 1993) although the specific details of findings differ. In the earliest study (Coulton et al., 1985) length of stay was not included in the regression equation but a bivariate correlation between length of stay and social work time expenditure was reported as being $r = .57$ compared with $r = .36$ for the current study.

Table 6.1
Summary of findings: utilisation of social work resources

Dependent variable	Relationship with independent variables
Total case costs	Length of stay
Total social work time costs	Length of stay (positive) Family disagreement: where discharged (positive) Income (inverse) Problems at work or school (positive)

In the study by Semke and colleagues (1993) length of stay, together with the other variables, accounted for 37% of the variance compared with 34% of variance in the current study. While these findings do not convey any meaning other than the longer patients are in hospital the more social work service they receive, length of stay is not satisfactory as an indicator of why some patients need more assistance then others. The purpose of this study was to find some other factors associated with use of social work resources.

The findings about the influence of income and disagreements with family about where the patient would go after leaving the hospital are consistent with the social work practice knowledge about the impact of having a lower socioeconomic status and the role of family members as important factors in discharge planning. A limited income reduces peoples' choices and it has been found to be associated with early re admission to hospital for elderly patients (Lockery et al., 1994). It is also expected that where there is conflict within the family discharge planning will be more difficult from the social worker's perspective (Abramson, 1990; Coulton, 1990; Proctor and Morrow-Howell, 1990; Rosenberg, 1994).

These factors were not identified as related to social work resource utilisation in the previous studies. Income level was not included in the study by Coulton and colleagues (1985) and in the other study (Semke et al., 1993) the variable of public assistance income or no income was not found to be significantly associated with increased use of resources.

Examination of cost drivers: Overview

There are some interesting questions arising from this data. The first issue relates to the hypotheses of the study. The intention was to obtain information about what drives costs in use of social work resources. To do this the intention was to do a thorough costing of social work services and if possible to compare a traditional costing (using variable costs and a proportion of fixed costs) with an activity based costing approach. The level of data required for this analysis was not made available. In the end the costing was similar to the product level costing as described by Cooper (1990) with identification of the variable costs that might be attached to the product, that is, the social work service provided to the patient.

In terms of product costing the majority of costs were from the social work time in service delivery. There were some additional costs from supervision time and professional study or training and a few patients received car parking subsidy. However, there is a question about the reliability and validity of the time and cost data collected. In the 1985 study (Coulton et al., 1985) social workers provided recording especially for the research team. For this study and the one in 1993 (Semke et al., 1993), the usual departmental recording system provided the data for service delivery time. For this study social workers were asked to provide additional information as well. It may be that busy social workers did not have time to provide accurate details, or they may not have been able to remember details of additional time spent in training or other activities, or how much time they spent in supervision discussing the particular case.

The difference in the findings when the dependent variable was changed confuses the information about resource utilisation to some degree. The consistency of the importance of length of stay is clear. It is also to be expected but it does not add information about the nature of the patient's condition or circumstances which might affect social work intervention.

Implications for social work practice

Within the managed care environment there is emphasis on brief and cost effective intervention (Brown et al., 1993; Cleary, 1994; Manheim and Feinglass, 1994; Tiesberg et al., 1994). The pressure to reduce costs in hospitals has increased over the last couple of years (Kayser et al., 1995; Morrisey, 1994) and so it is inevitable that these pressures within the hospital system have had an impact on social work practice (Berger et al., 1996; Poole, 1996). The effect of this can be seen in the results of this study.

The major finding in relation to social work practice is that so little time was spent on service delivery to patients that in many instances social workers would not have had an opportunity to achieve results while the patient was in hospital. With all patient oriented time accounted for this group of social workers reported seeing patients for a mean average time of less than two hours. This means that while some patients received social work input of some hours others received services for only minutes. Even considering many sources of inaccuracy in the recordings it is clear that social work input of time for most patients in this hospital at that time was brief.

Combined with this is the information that patients report having many problems after discharge. In spite of the inaccuracies that might arise in relation to their experiences while in the hospital it is likely that they were reporting their perceptions of the problems they experienced at the time of the interview. Given these findings there must be some question about whether it is best to locate social work resources within the hospital. It may be that social workers would be better placed in community centers providing follow up after discharge. This is not a proposition found in much social work literature to date. An analysis of the changing scene for hospital social workers identified some increase in services allocated to ambulatory or outpatient areas (Berger et al., 1996). Also there have been reports of social work services in community clinics (Resnick and Tighe, 1997) and calls for an increase in social work presence in primary health care settings (Berkman, 1996).

The data about disagreements experienced by patients from this study indicates that while quite a number of patients report having disagreements with hospital staff or with family most of these were minor and did not have a prolonged impact on the patient as they perceived the situation. This implies that there is no specific need for social work to target situations where there is disagreement except for the ten out of each hundred patients for whom the disagreement is a significant and disturbing event. Even then it is likely that those patients may be better served by social work intervention after discharge.

From the findings of the aspects of decision making this study suggests most patients in this group perceived themselves as having control over treatment and discharge planning decisions and that this was related to their satisfaction with decisions made while in the hospital. For whatever reason this hospital appears to deal with patients in a way which results in the patients perceiving themselves having as much control as is feasible given the circumstances, with only 10% of patients identifying some level of difficulty in control over decisions. This applies to both social work and non social work patients in this study and so it seems that it is not due to social work intervention. If other hospitals are likely to receive such a good report from patients then claims about the uncaring hospital system need to be examined more closely. The implication from this is that social workers do not need to be excessively worried that patients are having things done to them without consultation. At least this was the case for this hospital at the time of the study.

Implications for social work management

As has already been implied one of the issues arising from this study concerns allocation of social work resources. If the findings here were replicated in other studies there would be good reason to consider substantial reorganisation of social work services within health care. With the very short mean length of stay, patients have to deal with their illness and the recovery processes once they have left the hospital. The problems may well arise as they face issues of getting back to work and other daily routines. Social work services may be better located in community based facilities so as to be more accessible to patients and their families in the post discharge period.

If social workers are to be effective in the hospital setting then it would appear that it is important to structure service delivery so that there is a chance of providing benefit for the patients and their families. Some of the current service structures may be more geared toward administrative concerns. Social work departments may still feel that there is a need to prove the value of social work services by maintaining high visibility on wards by assessing as many patients as possible or by running high risk screening assessments. There may be good cause to question whether this provides services to help patients and families.

Some of the very short interventions may have been to assess whether someone identified by risk screening actually needed services. If high risk screening means that social workers must rush from patient to patient to do quick assessments then its value may need to be reviewed. This is especially so considering the inconsistent results in attempts to evaluate the effectiveness of such schemes (Coulton, 1988).

Whatever the motivation for the brief patient contact demonstrated for this group of social work patients there is cause to pause and consider what is being achieved by such patterns of service delivery that have become commonplace in so many hospitals. As an alternative to social workers assessing many patients and providing substantial services to a small proportion of the total number assessed there may be value in planning fewer hospital based assessments and more deliberate follow up into the community for some patients who may be more vulnerable because of the nature of the illness or their social circumstances. More extensive use of group services, particularly for outpatient clinics or in a community based center, may provide the means to provide the ongoing services that this group of patients indicate is warranted.

From quite another perspective the findings of this study raise issues about measurement and analysis of resource utilisation. The failure of this study to identify a number of meaningful factors which affect resource utilisation does not mean that other attempts will not succeed. As it stands the factors identified as cost drivers in this study, income and family disagreement in relation to discharge destination, may help managers to explore where there may be additional pressure on social work resources. At least the findings here may encourage managers to explore these issues further.

Implications for social work research

The decision making scales may require additional development and use before they can be used with confidence in analysis of the impact of the decision making environment on patients and family members. While the factor analysis produced the expected six factors and most items aligned in the same clusters as for the original study (Coulton et al., 1988) there were some variations with individual items and the internal consistency analysis produced some scales with alpha coefficients below .70. Given the continuing time pressure on patients and families within the health care system, the effort to monitor the decision making environment and its impact on satisfaction and outcomes is worth further study.

In many ways this study, like those before it (Coulton et al., 1988, 1989), has only commenced the examination of decision making processes in relation to service delivery. There is the potential for further studies which examine decision making by patients who have particular medical conditions. It may be that there are different decision making experiences according to the type of medical condition and the associated treatment. There is also the potential for further study of client decision making in other fields of social work endeavor with modification and development of decision making scales which may be used in a variety of settings.

There has been a special focus on disagreements as part of the decision making environment in this study. This particular group of patients have indicated that while they had a number of disagreements, especially with hospital staff, the experience was not necessarily difficult with long lasting impact on them. It would be interesting to test whether this is so for other groups of patients. The previous analyses of disagreements (Abramson et al., 1993) were from the social workers' perspective and this study has taken the patients' viewpoint. Future studies might combine examination of the social work, patient, family and hospital staff responses.

The difficulty with outcome measures remains a problem to be solved. While there is merit in attempting to measure problem reduction as an outcome for patients and families, future efforts at measurement of outcome need to ensure that social workers have had an opportunity to have an impact on the patient and family so that it is reasonable to expect that some change may have occurred in the person or in their situation and circumstances. It may be that the changes can be expected to last for only short periods of time (Grasso and Epstein, 1988; Sheldon, 1986) but there must be some evaluation of what is produced if continued funding for service delivery is to be obtained. There is much potential for a range of outcome studies which focus on specific programs of social work intervention and evaluation of effects at different points in time after intervention.

The difficulties in relation to analysis of the costs of social work services have been presented earlier. While this study failed to achieve a comprehensive costing of the social work service it must be considered in the context that this is a first attempt to apply activity based costing to social work services. Study in this field is in a very early stage of development and it is likely that additional research will produce more meaningful results. It may be that in order to obtain access to all the data needed the study needs to be undertaken from within the organisation. A partnership between an internal research group and an external management accounting academic may be the only way such studies will be completed. If funding can be obtained, studies in which recordings of time and costs are taken as they occur may provide more accurate and complete data than those which use existing workload statistics and accounting records. Whatever the arrangements or design many more studies which analyse the resources used in completion of social work service delivery will help to provide essential information for cost effectiveness analysis. The benefits to be obtained from cost analysis of social work services is not restricted to the hospital context. The application of activity based costing is relevant to the full range of human service contexts (Demone and Gibelman, 1989; Fein and Staff, 1991).

7 Summary

For many years social workers have been concerned about the effects of reduced length of hospital stay on patients and families (Kayser et al., 1995; Keigher, 1993; Reamer, 1985). There has been concern that the time pressured atmosphere of treatment reduces the patient's self determination in decision making about their treatment and plans for their future and contributes to problems experienced while in the hospital and after discharge. In association with this there has been previous research into the kinds of disagreements which occur between patients and hospital staff or family members about discharge planning (Abramson et al., 1993). There has also been study of decision making processes in relation to discharge planning (Coulton et al., 1988).

In another response to the pressures of the current health care system social workers have attempted to obtain a clearer understanding of social work productivity. In a small number of studies there has been examination of what factors contribute to increased use of social work resources (Coulton et al., 1985: Semke et al., 1993).

This study follows both strands of previous research. The first part examined the effect of the decision making environment on patients' satisfaction with decisions and on psychosocial outcomes. The second part attempted to identify the cost drivers for this sample of social work cases.

An exploratory survey design was used to compare the perceptions of 94 social work patients and 100 non social work patients about decision making and outcomes. The structured interview schedule by which data were collected in telephone interviews included the validated decision making scales developed by Coulton and colleagues (Coulton et al., 1988), and other questions developed specifically for this study. Patients were asked to rate themselves at the time of the interview and at the time when they were in the hospital in relation to a list of psychosocial problems derived from the Hospital Social Work Directors productivity measurement system (Keller et al., 1993).

For the analysis of cost drivers the recordings of social work time spent in service delivery were combined with social work reports about time in supervision, training or other activities required in providing services to each patient. This social work time data was translated into dollars using information about salary costs for each individual worker. Information about other costs was also collected and for the most part this was restricted to parking subsidy costs for a small number of patients.

It was hypothesised that aspects which facilitate decision making, that is, certainty about outcomes, control over decisions, and family support, would be associated with higher levels of patient satisfaction with decisions and better psychosocial outcomes. Factors which inhibit decision making, namely, hypervigilance, having restricted choices, being rushed, and having disagreements were expected to be inversely related to psychosocial outcomes. It was also hypothesised that the outcomes would be better for social work as compared with non social work patients. The final hypothesis was that disagreements and types and number of problems would increase the cost of social work services provided.

The first issue to arise was the difficulty in obtaining the data. More than half the patients approached to participate in the study were not able or chose not to be part of the project. While a proportion were excluded for good reason in that they were not able to communicate or were too ill there were many non participators who did not provide a reason. This high attrition rate causes doubts about the representativeness of this sample and so any suggestions from the data must be treated as indicators for further research.

Multiple regression analysis was used to test all hypotheses. The findings were not as anticipated. In relation to the decision making environment the facilitator aspects of certainty and control, but not family support, were found to be associated with higher ratings of satisfaction with decisions made while in the hospital. This finding must be considered in the context of the factor analysis results which failed to replicate the structure of the decision making scales. Another cause for concern is that the data were not normally distributed and most patients reported high satisfaction with decisions, feeling that they had sufficient control over decision making, high levels of family support and a satisfactory level of certainty about outcomes.

The attempt to use patient ratings of problems at the time of the interview and when they were in the hospital as a post/then measure of change in level in problem severity did not work as intended. About a third of the patients were recorded as experiencing little or no change in the level of problems from time of being in the hospital to the time of the interview. Another third did show an improvement in their situation. That is, about a third of the patients described themselves as having fewer and/or less severe problems at the time of interview. The rest of the patients indicated that they had an increase in problems after discharge. In addition there were no significant differences between the social work and non social work patients in terms of changes in the problem scores.

When the problems score at the time of the interview was used as the outcome measure it was found that social work patients had a significantly higher problem score than non social work patients at the time of the interview.

In the examination of disagreements between patients and hospital staff or with family members the findings were that almost half of the patients, both social work and non social work patients experienced disagreements with hospital staff. However, most of these patients also reported that the disagreement had not had a significant impact on them. Approximately 90% of patients stated that any disagreement that had occurred had not made the time in the hospital and planning for the future more difficult for them. Disagreements with family members were less common, particularly for non social work patients, and the impact of those disagreements too appeared minimal.

In relation to utilisation of social work resources the most important finding was that social workers are able to spend very little time with patients and families. The cost drivers identified in this study included length of stay in hospital, lower income level and the existence of family disagreement about discharge destination.

The contribution of this study

In relation to the decision making environment and the concerns about limitations on client self determination the results of this study indicate that most patients do not have a concern about impediments to their participation in decision making. While there are limitations to this study and some concerns about the validity of the decision making scales used, the responses and the statistical analysis indicate that for this group of people there was sufficient information, time and choice in making decisions. Given that about 90% of this sample indicated that they had as much control over decisions as they wished, there may be room for social workers to be somewhat less anxious about how other hospital staff respond to patients. If this finding were replicated in other situations than it may be considered safe for social work intervention to be targeted toward other issues for the patient and their family.

The importance of this study is not so much from the results of the analysis of the impact of the decision making environment as from the information about the pattern of problems experienced by patients and the patterns of social work intervention. Putting together the information that social workers spent a mean of less than 2 hours per patient, and that a considerable proportion of this group of patients experienced a higher degree of problems at the time of the interview than when they were in the hospital, there is good cause to reconsider where social workers might be strategically placed to provide the optimal service. The shape of the social work service might be geared less toward assessment and more toward sufficient time per patient spent in group work, or in individual and family work with a smaller number of patients who are identified as requiring ongoing services. This study raises this issue for further examination.

Finally, this study has attempted to use an approximation of activity based costing to examine influences on costs of social work services. This is the first contribution of publicly available data about cost drivers which translates resources into dollars. This study shows that even if there are limitations on the availability of the data it is worth doing because of the potential value of the information to be derived from such analyses. The results from this study, which identify patient's income level, the existence of family disagreements about discharge destination, and length of stay in hospital as the costs drivers, are not of major importance as final results. These results are derived from a very small sample of social work cases in one hospital. Perhaps other studies in other settings may add to the picture.

It is important that this study is a first attempt at cost analysis in a framework which attempts to identify the actual costs which might be attributable to the work with each patient. The use of activity based costing in place of measures of productivity which rely on social work time or on costs in terms of standard cost per social work hour has much to offer in examination of what our services use in resources. Use of activity based costing, which requires effort to trace costs from work activities to the product or service, does have the potential to give more accurate understanding of how resources are used and which factors are associated with increase use of social work resources. If a number of studies using an activity based costing framework were undertaken, the cumulative information about cost drivers may well provide valuable information about resource requirements for services in relation to particular patient or client groups.

Directions for future research

The decision making scales used in this study may require further development if they are to be used confidently to measure the decision making environment for patients. Additional items for all dimensions and a repeated confirmatory factor analysis may be needed. Another potential development is in relation to decision making by family members. Particularly in the acute care setting when the patient may be too ill to be an active participant, family decision makers may be relied upon by both the patient and the hospital system.

The importance of disagreements between patients and others may be more important in other settings than shown in this hospital and for this group of patients. Further study from the patient's viewpoint, and study which compares the patient, family and hospital staff viewpoints may clarify whether this area has significant impact on patient care. From this study the indication is that other aspects of the patient and family situation may be more important than the disagreements which may not have a long term impact.

Certainly there is encouragement from examination of this group of patients to examine further what happens to patients after they leave the hospital. The use of problem ratings to measure outcomes for patients has potential but must be used in a context where social workers have a realistic opportunity to have an impact on the client's situation.

While many in the profession may question the value or wisdom of undertaking this exercise the view taken here is that social workers must take responsibility to do their own analysis of costs and productivity. It is too important to be left to the accountants. If social work cannot show that it is cost effective then the profession will struggle to survive. Costing information, identification of cost drivers connected to outcome data, has much to offer in equipping social workers to analyse their work. The use of activity based costing provides a framework for this type of research that is understandable and usable for social work practitioners. This kind of data may help to refine and improve work practices and to maintain a focus on the effectiveness of social work intervention. The ultimate beneficiaries will be the patients and their families.

Appendix A

Data collection forms

Data From Hospital Records

Patient ID.   Location: zip code

Address:

Admission date: Telephone number:

Discharge date:

Age: Gender:

Marital Status:

Medical Service:

DRG:

Readmission date:

Discharge Date 2:

Social Work Time Expenditure

To:

I am writing to you about one of your patients who was recently discharged. The information requested here is part of the research program "social work services and patient decision making" which is one of the research projects being conducted in the Social Work Services Department. It would be helpful if you could complete the following information and leave the form in my pigeon-hole. If I do not receive this form I will understand that the only social work time expenditure for this patient was recorded in the workload statistics available through the patient inquiry system. Thank you for taking the time to help with this data collection. If you have any questions please ask Director of Social Work or give me a call on 962 0414.

Patricia Hansen

Patient ID: Patient Name:

Time spent in work with patient and family. This information is in the stats system. Only enter it here if the time is different to what is in the stats.
_____hours_____minutes

Time spent in supervision discussing
patient_____hours_____minutes

Time spent in training or in reading professional literature in last month on topic relevant to patient_____hours_____minutes

Has there been any other special activity or expenditure of time or resources for this patient and family? _____

_____

Have you any other comments about the resources required to assist this patient and family? _____

_____

Thank you very much for your assistance.

Parking Subsidy: Yes   No

Time of tickets: Amount of subsidy: $_____

Appendix B

Letter to patients

Dear

My name is Patricia Hansen. I am associated with the Social Work Department at the hospital in a research project on how patients make decisions about treatment and plans for the future. The aim of this research is to learn more about how patients are involved in making decisions/treatment plans and to understand what helps and hinders patients in making decisions.

You have been selected to participate in this study because you have recently been discharged from the hospital. The study involves a telephone interview that takes approximately 30 minutes. All information is kept in strict confidence. If at any time during this study you have problems with the way the research is being conducted please contact the Director of Social Work (617- 932 - 6469).

In two weeks I will call you to answer any questions you may have and to see if you are willing to participate. A postcard is enclosed for you to return to let us know if you do not wish to receive a call.

Your participation is completely voluntary but it is important for us to to talk with as many patients as possible for scientific validity. I hope you will consider being part of this study.

Sincerely,

Patricia Hansen
Research Associate

Postcard

I do not wish to be a participant in your   Director, Social Work Services
study of social work services and patient
decision making.

Appendix C

Interview schedule

My name is Patricia Hansen and I am calling with regard to the hospital Social Work Department survey on patient decision-making. We are interested in how you perceive the way decisions were made about treatment and plans for the future while you were in hospital. We want to use this information to improve services provided to patients at the hospital. This interview will take 30 minutes. If you do not understand any question please ask me to explain. You may refuse to answer any question.

Patient ID: Location:

Telephone number:

In this first section we want to obtain some basic details about you?

1. How many years of education have you completed?

2. What is your current marital status?   2a. Gender: 0 Male

Single	Separated/divorced	1 Female
Married/Partner	Widowed	

3. Which is closest to the yearly income for your household? Could you tell me when I say the one that is right for you.

Less than $10,000	$50,000 - $69,999
$10,000 - $29,999	$70,000 - $89,999
$30,000 - $ 49,999	$90,000 and over

4.	Which is the closest to the group that describes your ethnic background?
African-American
American native
Asian-American
European origin. Specify if relevant to person interviewed.
Hispanic/Latino
Other: specify

5.	Do you live alone or with other people?
5.1	Alone
(If respondent lives with other people) How are they related to you?
Response given by patient will be coded in the following categories
5.2	Patient and spouse/ partner only
5.3	Patient, spouse/partner and children
5.4	Patient and children only
5.5	Patient and others who have formed a new family (e.g. stepchildren)
5.6	Many generations of family living in the same house
5.7	Patient with friends who have become so close that they are like family
5.8	Group living with no close relationship with other people in the household
5.9	Other, specify

6.	When you were in hospital were you seen by a social worker?
	0 No			1 Yes
6.1	For how long did you see the social worker? (Respondent will be asked how often and whether they can estimate in terms of number of times)
6.2	From the time you were admitted to hospital have you seen another social worker apart from the one you saw at hospital?
	0 No			1 Yes
	Do you mind telling me who that social worker is ?(which agency).

In this part we have a series of statements describing aspects of making decisions. During a stay in hospital it is often necessary for patients to make decisions about treatment and their care after leaving the hospital. I would like you to think about when you were in the hospital and to respond to each statement in terms of whether it was true for you when you were in the hospital. After each statement I will read the scale to you.

Scale:	Not at all true			1
	Somewhat true			2
	Half true and half false	3
	Mostly true			4
	Completely true			5

105

| 7. | I felt my situation was pretty hopeless. | 1 | 2 | 3 | 4 | 5 |

| 8. | I worried a lot about what would happen. | 1 | 2 | 3 | 4 | 5 |

| 9. | I was afraid of what would happen to me after leaving the hospital. | 1 | 2 | 3 | 4 | 5 |

10. I felt I had to decide quickly. 1 2 3 4 5

11. I thought a great deal about what to do. 1 2 3 4 5

12. It was hard to tell what was going to happen. 1 2 3 4 5

13. Everyone tried to tell me what to do. 1 2 3 4 5

14. My family supported my thinking on. this. 1 2 3 4 5

15. I felt my family would accept my decision. 1 2 3 4 5

16. It was clear what my family thought was best. 1 2 3 4 5

17. I just looked at this one choice of plan. 1 2 3 4 5

18. This was the only plan I looked at. 1 2 3 4 5

19. This seems like a final decision. 1 2 3 4 5

20. I was fairly certain about how I would do after leaving the hospital. 1 2 3 4 5

21. I always knew something could be worked out. 1 2 3 4 5

22. I had enough information about my condition to decide what to do. 1 2 3 4 5

23.	I knew what the doctor thought I should do.	1	2	3	4	5
24.	I knew the choice was up to me.	1	2	3	4	5
25.	I had the final say about the decision.	1	2	3	4	5
26.	Everyone seemed quite rushed.	1	2	3	4	5
27.	I had little time to decide.	1	2	3	4	5

When decisions need to be made it is not uncommon for there to be disagreements among the people involved. For example, there might be disagreement between a patient and doctor or between a patient and a family member. The next few questions are about the disagreements you may have had with others while in hospital and how you felt about the decisions that were made.

28. When you were in hospital how often did you disagree with a doctor, nurse, social worker or other health care providers about treatment or plans for the future?

   1 Not at all
   2 Rarely
   3 Sometimes
   4 Quite a bit
   5 Often
   6 All of the time

29. Were the disagreements about:

29.1 what kind of treatment you would receive   0 No   1 Yes

29.2 the treatment that had been given to you   0 No   1 Yes

29.3 the services (food, accommodation etc) provided at the hospital
                                                       0 No   1 Yes

29.4 when you would be discharged   0 No   1 Yes

29.5 where you would go after leaving hospital   0 No   1 Yes

29.6 what treatment you would receive after leaving hospital

                                                              0 No   1 Yes

29.7 other issues, specifically   0 No   1 Yes

30. When you were in hospital how often did you disagree with family members about your treatment, plans for the future or other decisions?

    1 Not at all
    2 Rarely
    3 Sometimes
    4 Quite a bit
    5 Often
    6 All of the time

31. Were the disagreements about:

31.1 the treatment you were having   0 No   1 Yes

31.2 who would manage your home and responsibilities (home, children/parents/relatives, work, business, finances) while you were in hospital

                                                               0 No   1 Yes

31.3 your home and responsibilities not being looked after properly while you were in hospital   0 No   1 Yes

31.4 who would look after you after you left hospital   0 No   1 Yes

31.5 where you would go after you left hospital   0 No   1 Yes

31.6 continuation of disagreements that you had with your family before you were in hospital   0 No   1 Yes

31.7 other issues, specifically   0 No   1 Yes

32. How satisfied are you now with the decisions you made then?

Scale:

Not at all satisfied	1	Quite satisfied	4
Not very satisfied	2	Very satisfied	5
Somewhat satisfied	3	Completely satisfied	6

In this next part we want to find out how things worked out for you in hospital and afterwards.

33. What problems are important to you right now? I will read out a list of problems and ask you how serious each one is for you right now. A problem is a serious one if you think that something should be done about it.

Scale:

Not at all serious	1	Quite serious	4
Not very serious	2	Very serious	5
Somewhat serious	3	Extremely serious	6

33.1   Accommodation   1   2   3   4   5   6

33.2   Financial issues   1   2   3   4   5   6

33.3   Adjusting to the illness and
        treatment   1   2   3   4   5   6

33.4   Helping the family and close friends to adjust to the illness and treatment
                                                               1   2   3   4   5   6

33.5   Family relationship problems
                                                               1   2   3   4   5   6

33.6   Relationship problems with other people (not family)
                                                               1   2   3   4   5   6

33.7   Emotional problems   1   2   3   4   5   6

33.8   Problems about work or
        school   1   2   3   4   5   6

33.9   Legal problems   1   2   3   4   5   6

33.10   Other problems   1   2   3   4   5   6

34.   Thinking back to when you were in hospital what were the major problems for you?

Scale:

Not at all serious	1	Quite serious	4
Not very serious	2	Very serious	5
Somewhat serious	3	Extremely serious	6

34.1.   Accommodation   1   2   3   4   5   6

Who helped you with your accommodation problems (Help not needed, No-one, Doctor, Nurse, Social Worker, Family Member, other   )

34.2   Financial problems   1   2   3   4   5   6

Who helped you with your financial problems (Help not needed, No-one, Doctor, Nurse, Social Worker, Family Member,
other   )

34.3   Adjusting to the illness and treatment   1   2   3   4   5   6

Who helped you with your adjustment problems (Help not needed, No-one, Doctor, Nurse, Social Worker, Family Member, other   )

34.4   Helping the family and close friends adjust to the illness and treatment
                                         1   2   3   4   5   6

Who helped you with your family's adjustment problems (Help not needed, No-one, Doctor, Nurse, Social Worker, Family Member, other   )

34.5   Family relationship problems
                                         1   2   3   4   5   6

Who helped you with your family relationship problems (Help not needed, No-one, Doctor, Nurse, Social Worker, Family Member, other   )

34.6   Relationship problems with other people (not family)
                                         1   2   3   4   5   6

Who helped you with your relationship problems with others (Help not needed, No-one, Doctor, Nurse, Social Worker, Family Member, other   )

34.7   Emotional problems   1   2   3   4   5   6

Who helped you with your emotional problems (Help not needed, No-one, Doctor, Nurse, Social Worker, Family Member, other   )

34.8   Problems about work or school   1   2   3   4   5   6

Who helped you with your school or work problems (Help not needed, No-one, Doctor, Nurse, Social Worker, Family Member, other   )

34.9   Legal problems.   1   2   3   4   5   6

Who helped you with your legal problems (Help not needed, No-one, Doctor, Nurse, Social Worker, Family Member, other   )

34.10   Other problems.   1   2   3   4   5   6

Who helped you with your legal problems (Help not needed, No-one, Doctor, Nurse, Social Worker, Family Member, other   )

In these last questions we would like you to comment in your own words on the decisions you made while you were in hospital.

35.   Did you have as much control as you wanted over the decisions about your treatment and plans for the future? How did you get that control? Was it hard to get control over decisions?

36.   Did the disagreements that occurred make being in hospital and planning for the future more difficult for you? How?

37.   Have you any other comments you would like to make?

Thank you very much for your participation in this study.

Appendix D

Tables of results

Table 4.5

Correlation matrix, means and standard deviations of decision making scales (n = 194)

				Variables		
Variables Mean(SD)	1	2	3	4	5	
1. Hypervigilance 1.960(.763)						
2. Family Support 4.287(.993)	-.014					
3. Restricted Choice 3.192(1.418)	.004	.017				
4. Certainty 4.066(.858)	-.367***	.161*	.047			
5. Control 4.366(.972)	-.217**	.206**	-.068	.406***		
6. Rushed 1.933(1.211)	.473***	-.092	.146*	-.314***	-.186**	

* p < .05, ** p < .01, ***p < .001

Table 4.13
Distribution of helpers identified by social work and non social work patients
(n = 192)

Identified Helper	SW (n = 94) n(%)	NSW (n = 98) n(%)	Total n(%)
Family	26 (28%)	28 (29%)	54 (28%)
None	19 (20%)	16 (16%)	35 (18%)
Others	17 (18%)	14 (14%)	31 (16%)
Nurse	13 (14%)	10 (10%)	23 (12%)
Social Worker	17 (18%)	0 (0%)	17 (9%)
Doctor	7 (7%)	8 (8%)	15 (8%)
Social Worker and others	12 (13%)	0 (0%)	12 (6%)
Everybody	5 (5%)	4 (4%)	9 (5%)

Table 4.14
Number of problems when in hospital for social work
and non social work patients
(n = 190)

Problems in Hospital	SW n(%)	NSW n(%)	Total n(%)
No problems	23 (24%)	36 (37%)	59 (31%)
One problem only	26 (28%)	23 (24%)	49 (26%)
Two problems	20 (21%)	23 (24%)	43 (23%)
Three problems	10 (11%)	7 (7%)	17 (9%)
Four problems	11 (12%)	3 (3%)	14 (7%)
Five problems	0 (0%)	3 (3%)	3 (2%)
Six problems	3 (3%)	1 (1%)	4 (2%)
Seven problems	1 (1%)	0 (0%)	1 (0%)
Total	94 (100%)	96 (100%)*	190 (100%)*

* Variation in total percentage due to rounding

Table 4.15
Number of problems at time of interview for social work
and non social work patients
(n = 190)

Problems in Hospital	SW n(%)	NSW n(%)	Total n(%)
No problems	24 (25%)	45 (47%)	69 (36%)
One problem only	10 (11%)	22 (23%)	32 (17%)
Two problems	23 (24%)	10 (10%)	33 (17%)
Three problems	15 (16%)	9 (9%)	24 (13%)
Four problems	9 (10%)	4 (4%)	13 (7%)
Five problems	6 (6%)	4 (4%)	10 (5%)
Six problems	4 (4%)	2 (2%)	6 (3%)
Seven problems	0 (0%)	0 (0%)	0 (0%)
Eight problems	3 (3%)	0 (0%)	3 (2%)
Total	94 (100%)*	96 (100%)*	190 (100%)

* Variation in total percentage due to rounding

Table 4.16
Distribution of problems scores at time of interview for
social work and non social work patients
(n = 190)

Problems in Hospital	SW n(%)	NSW n(%)	Total n(%)
No score	23 (24%)	45 (47%	68 (36%)
1 - 10	47 (50%)	38 (39%)	85 (45%)
11 - 20	19 (20%)	10 (10%)	29 (15%)
21 - 30	3 (3%)	3 (3%)	6 (3%)
31 - 40	2 (2%)	0 (0%)	2 (1%)
41 - 50	0 (0%)	0 (0%)	0 (0%)
51 - 60	0 (0%)	0 (0%)	0 (0%)
Total	94 (100%)*	96 (100%)*	190 (100%)

* Variation in total percentage due to rounding

Table 4.17
Distribution of problem scores when in the hospital for social work and non social work patients (n = 190)

Problems in Hospital	SW n(%)	NSW n(%)	Total n(%)
No Score	23 (24%)	36 (37%)	59 (31%)
1 - 10	53 (56%)	49 (51%)	102 (54%)
11 - 20	15 (16%)	10 (10%)	25 (13%)
21 - 30	2 (2%)	1 (1%)	3 (2%)
31 - 40	1 (1%)	0 (0%)	1 (0%)
41 -50	0 (0%)	0 (0%)	0 (%)
51 - 60	0 (0%)	0 (0%)	0 (0%)
Total	94 (100%)*	96 (100%)*	190 (100%)*

* Variation in total percentage due to rounding

Table 4.18
Differences in problem scores (then - now) for
social work and non social work patients (n = 190)

Problems in Hospital	SW n(%)	NSW n(%)	Total n(%)
Minus 20 to minus 11	6 (6%)	1 (1%)	7 (4%)
Minus 10 to minus 1	33 (35%)	26 (27%)	59 (31%)
Zero	21 (22%)	38 (40%)	59 (31%)
Plus 1 to plus 10	32 (34%)	27 (28%)	59 (31%)
Plus 11 to plus 20	2 (2%)	3 (3%)	5 (3%)
Plus 21 to plus 30	0 (0%)	1 (1%)	1 (1%)
Total	94 (100%)*	96 (100%)	190 (100%)*

* Variation in total percentage due to rounding

Table 4.20

Correlation matrix, means and standard deviations of selected independent variables and dependent variable satisfaction with decisions (n = 193)

Variables Mean(SD)		Variables					
	1	2	3	4	5	6	7
1. Control 4.368(.975)							
2. Certainty 4.062(.859)	.408***						
3. Family 4.283(.994)	.208**	.158*					
4. Age 51.622(16.661)	.077	.052	.075				
5. Marital Status .570(.496)	.060	.087	.322***	.024			
6. Gender .648(.429)	.101	.057	.036	-.108	.017		
7. Ethnicity .762(.427)	.118	.073	.160**	.028	.054	-.082	
8. Education 14.422 (2.780)	-.028	-.099	.018	-.088	.153*	-.040	-.018
9. Gap 44.922(15.373)	.097	.088	.109	-.040	.082	-.039	.095
10. Length of Stay 8.254 (7.182)	-.095	-.016	.120*	.002	.129	-.081	.033
11. Category: Social Work .487(.501)	.068	-.059	-.087	-.086	-.096	.046	-.039
Satisfaction/ Decisions 5.238(1.223)	.343***	.422***	.150*	.173**	.007	.011	.179**

table continues

121

Table 4.20 continued

Correlation matrix, means and standard deviations of selected independent variables and dependent variable satisfaction with decisions (n = 193)

Variables Mean(SD)	Variables			
	8	9	10	11
9. Gap 44.922(15.373)	.081			
10. Length of Stay 8.254(7.182)	-.085	-.191**		
11. Category: Social Work .487(.501)	-.057	-.487***	.075	
Satisfaction/ Decisions 5.238(1.223)	-.093	.039	.010	-.071

* p < .05, ** p < .01, *** p < .001

Table 4.22

Correlation matrix, means and standard deviations of selected independent variables and dependent variable satisfaction with decisions: non social work patients (n = 99)

Variables Mean(SD)	Variables						
	1	2	3	4	5	6	7
1. Control 4.303(1.054)							
2. Certainty 4.111(.827)	.467***						
3. Family 4.367(.957)	.224*	.132					
4. Age 53.020(16.379)	-.004	.141	.030				
5. Marital Status .616(.489)	.010	.119	.297***	-.040			
6. Gender .626(.486)	.193*	.250**	.057	-.150	.120		
7. Ethnicity .778(.418)	.143	.168*	.053	.025	-.022	-.112	
8. Education 14.576(2.882)	.009	-.074	-.002	-.150	.166	-.034	.053
9. Gap 52.202(9.984)	.266**	.200*	.190*	-.117	-.028	.037	.170
10. Length of Stay 7.727(7.023)	-.211*	-.099	.044	.000	.142	-.141	-.021
Satisfaction/ Decisions 5.323(1.194)	.379***	.573***	.133	.099	-.030	-.087	.289**

table continues

123

Table 4.22 continued

Correlation matrix, means and standard deviations of selected independent variables and dependent variable satisfaction with decisions: non social work patients (n = 99)

Variables Mean(SD)	Variables		
	8	9	10
9. Gap 52.202(9.984)	.078		
10. Length of Stay 7.727(7.023)	-.139	-.226*	
Satisfaction/ Decisions 5.323(1.194)	-.200*	.076	.018

* p < .05, ** p < .01, *** p < .001

Table 4.24

Correlation matrix, means and standard deviations of selected independent variables and dependent variable satisfaction with decisions: social work patients (n = 94)

		Variables						
Variables	*Mean(SD)*	1	2	3	4	5	6	7
1. Control	4.436(.884)							
2. Certainty	4.011(.893)	.359***						
3. Family	4.195(1.030)	.209*	.174*					
4. Age	50.149(16.915)	.191*	-.041	.103				
5. Marital Status	.521(.502)	.136	.047	.335***	.072			
6. Gender	.670(.473)	-.025	-.132	.023	-.057	-.083		
7. Ethnicity	.745(.438)	.096	-.020	.254**	.025	.123	-.047	
8. Education	14.261(2.674)	-.070	-.134	.030	-.032	.130	-.042	.053
9. Gap	37.255(16.342)	.076	-.009	.012	-.084	.086	-.057	.039
10. Length of Stay	8.809(7.342)	.032	.069	.205*	.017	.132	-.028	.092
Satisfaction/ Decisions	5.149(1.253)	.320***	.277**	.155	.234*	.029	-.061	.070

table continues

125

Table 4.24 continued

Correlation, means and standard deviations of selected independent variables and dependent variable satisfaction with decisions: social work patients (n = 94)

Variables	Mean(SD)	Variables		
		8	9	10
9. Gap	37.255(16.342)	.054		
10. Length of Stay	8.809(7.342)	-.018	-.153	
Satisfaction/ Decisions	5.149(1.253)	.014	-.039	.014

* p < .05, ** p < .01, *** p < .001

Table 4.26

Correlation matrix, means and standard deviations of selected independent variables and dependent variable problem difference scores (n = 190)

			Variables				
Variables Mean(SD)	1	2	3	4	5	6	7
1. Control 4.368(.981)							
2. Certainty 4.058(.863)	.408***						
3. Family 4.275(.999)	.208**	.154*					
4. Age 51.500(16.622)	.080	.045	.068				
5. Category .495(.501)	.069	-.054	-.080	-.081			
6. Education 14.413(2.784)	-.028	-.106	.013	-.106	-.054		
7. Marital Status .574(.496)	.064	.098	.334***	.041	-.105	.169**	
8. Gender .653(.477)	.094	.055	.039	-.103	.037	-.039	.019
9. Ethnicity .763(.426)	.115	.077	.166*	.047	-.043	-.004	.045
10. Gap 44.700(15.379)	.097	.081	.102	-.051	-.480***	.075	.096
11. Length of Stay 8.305(7.227)	-.095	-.014	.124*	.005	.069	-.084	.127*
Problem Difference -.558(5.564)	-.008	.122*	.200**	.007	-.124*	.002	.155*

table continues

Table 4.26 continued

Correlation matrix, means and standard deviations of selected independent variables and dependent variable problem difference scores (n = 190)

Variables Mean(SD)	Variables			
	8	9	10	11
9. Ethnicity .763(.426)	-.094			
10. Gap 44.700(15.379)	-.033	.102		
11. Length of Stay 8.305(7.227)	-.087	.032	-.186	
Problem Difference -.558(5.564)	.142*	.002	.016	.115

* p < .05, ** p < .01, *** p < .001

128

Table 4.28

Correlation matrix, means and standard deviations of selected independent variables and dependent variable log problems scores at the time of the interview (n = 122)

Variables Mean(SD)				*Variables*			
	1	2	3	4	5	6	7
1. Control 4.303(1.009)							
2. Certainty 3.887(.904)	.442***						
3. Family 4.205(.974)	.243**	.132					
4. Age 49.467(16.044)	.126	.011	.068				
5. Category .582(.495)	.099	.042	-.072	-.158*			
6. Education 14.439(2.896)	-.049	-.153*	.010	-.055	-.050		
7. Marital Status .533(.501)	.111	.042	.288***	.100	-.028	.094	
8. Gender .598(.492)	.056	.000	-.068	-.040	.119	-.020	.004
9. Ethnicity .762(.427)	.025	-.016	.138	-.025	-.083	.001	.056
10. Gap 44.459(16.265)	.125	.037	.169*	-.033	-.425***	.094	.108
11. Length of Stay 7.795(6.855)	-.104	-.076	.138	.015	-.079	-.097	.102
Problems Now 1.791(.866)	-.086	-.163*	-.234**	-.206*	.228**	.134	-.116

table continues

Table 4.28 continued

Correlation matrix, means and standard deviations of selected independent variables and dependent variable problem scores at the time of the interview (n = 122)

Variables Mean(SD)	*Variables*			
	8	9	10	11
9. Ethnicity .762(.427)	-.143			
10. Gap 44.459(16.265)	-.092	.116		
11. Length of Stay 7.795(6.855)	-.164*	.006	-.118	
Problems Now 1.791(.866)	.064	-.120	.018	-.131

* p < .05, ** p < .01, *** p < .001

Table 4.30

Correlation matrix, means and standard deviations of selected independent variables and dependent variable problem difference scores (n = 190)

Variables Mean(SD)	Variables						
	1	2	3	4	5	6	7
1. Hypervigilance 1.956(.764)							
2. Restricted 3.179(1.418)	-.002						
3. Rushed 1.913(1.203)	.469***	.126*					
4. Hospital Disagree .937(1.352)	.367***	-.061	.347***				
5. Family Disagree .321(.815)	.292***	-.047	.102	.105			
6. Age 51.500(16.622)	-.255***	.143*	-.207	-.176**	-.104		
7. Category .495(.501)	.244***	.026	.098	.046	.075	-.081	
8. Marital Status .574(.496)	-.009	-.069	-.031	.023	-.118	.041	-.105
9. Gender .653(.477)	.072	-.103	.067	-.034	.003	-.103	.037
10. Ethnicity .763(.426)	-.090	-.023	-.123*	-.054	-.191**	.047	-.043
11. Education 14.413(2.784)	.040	.031	.176**	.081	-.039	-.106	-.054
12. Gap 44.700(15.379)	-.046	.043	.003	-.048	-.097	-.051	-.480***
13. Length of Stay 8.305(7.227)	.064	.017	.028	.131*	-.025	.005	.069
Problem Difference -.558(5.564)	-.035	.017	.130*	.035	-.026	.007	-.124*

table continues

131

Table 4.30 continued

Correlation matrix, means and standard deviations of selected independent variables and dependent variable problem difference scores (n = 190)

Variables Mean(SD)		Variables				
	8	9	10	11	12	13
9. Gender .653(.477)	.019					
10. Ethnicity .763(.426)	.045	-.094				
11. Education 14.413(2.784)	.169**	-.039	-.004			
12. Gap 44.700(15.379)	.096	-.033	.102	.075		
13. Length of Stay 8.305(7.227)	.127*	-.087	.032	-.084	-.186**	
Problem Difference -.558(5.564)	.155*	.142*	.002	.002	.016	.115

* p < .05, ** p < .01, *** p < .001

132

Table 4.32

Correlation matrix, means and standard deviations of selected independent variables and dependent variable log problems at the time of the interview (n = 122)

Variables Mean(SD)		1	2	3	4	5	6	7
					Variables			
1. Hypervigilance 2.114(.779)								
2. Restricted 3.164(1.382)		-.055						
3. Rushed 2.061(1.231)		.490***	.190*					
4. Hospital Disagreement 1.172(1.487)		.354***	-.071	.342***				
5. Family Disagreement .451(.972)		.286***	-.062	.087	.043			
6. Age 49.467(16.044)		-.215**	.079	-.145	-.158*	-.077		
7. Category .582(.495)		.179*	.016	.124	.042	.051	-.158	
8. Education 14.439(2.896)		.028	.112	.086	.004	-.055	-.055	.050
9. Marital Status .533(.501)		.019	-.071	-.100	.053	-.124	.100	-.028
10. Gender .598(.492)		.132	-.153*	.157	-.006	.036	-.040	.119
11. Ethnicity .762(.427)		-.060	.062	-.043	-.065	-.257**	-.025	.083
12. Gap 44.459(16.265)		.008	.048	.029	-.083	-.124	-.033	.425***
13. Length of Stay 7.795(6.855)		.116	.061	.079	.221**	.005	.015	-.079
Log Problems Now 1.791(.866)		.329***	-.142	.055	.209***	.223**	-.206*	.228**

table continues

133

Table 4.32 continued

Correlation matrix, means and standard deviations of selected independent variables and dependent variable log problems at the time of the interview (n = 122)

Variables Mean(SD)			Variables					
	8	9	10	11	12	13		
9. Marital Status .533(.501)	.094							
10. Gender .598(.492)	-.020	.004						
11. Ethnicity .762(.427)	.001	.056	-.143					
12. Gap 44.459(16.265)	.094	.108	-.092	.116				
13. Length of Stay 7.7795(6.855)	-.097	.102	-.164*	.006	-.118			
Log Problems Now 1.791(.866)	.134	-.116	.064	-.120	.018	-.131		

* p < .05, ** p < .01, *** p < .001

134

Table 5.4

Correlation matrix, means and standard deviations of selected independent variables and dependent variable total case costs (n = 77)

Variables _Mean(SD)_	1	2	3	4	5	6	7
				Variables			
1. Length of stay 8.455(7.170)							
Hospital disagreements:							
2. When discharged .182(.388)	-.077						
3. Where discharge .091(.289)	-.014	.202*					
Family disagreements:							
4. Who cares for .091(.289)	-.077	.202*	.214*				
5. Where discharge .026(.160)	.116	.135	.232*	.232*			
6. Number problems	-.101	.159	.121	.175	.167		
7. Income 2.727(1.392)	.101	-.077	.128	-.330**	.091	.071	

table continues

Table 5.4 continued

Correlation matrix, means and standard deviations of selected independent variables and dependent variable total case costs (n = 77)

Variables Mean(SD)	1	2	3	4	5	6	7
				Variables			
8. Ethnicity .779(.417)	.157	.089	.168	-.050	-.110	-.122	.167
Total case costs 56.259(68.806)	.297**	.189*	.012	.172	.186	.099	-.134

Variables Mean(SD)	8
	Variables
Total case costs 56.259(68.806)	.041

* p < .05, ** p < .01, *** p < .001

136

Table 5.6

Correlation matrix, means and standard deviations of selected independent variables and dependent variable total social work time costs (n = 77)

		Variables						
Variables Mean(SD)		1	2	3	4	5	6	7
1. Length of stay 8.455(7.170)								
Hospital disagreements:								
2. When discharged .182(.388)		-.077						
3. Where discharge .091(.289)		-.014	.202*					
Family disagreements:								
4. Who care for .091(.289)		-.077	.202*	.214*				
5. Where discharge .026(.160)		.116	.135	.232*	.232*			
6. Number problems 1.792(1.681)		-.101	.159	.121	.175	.167		
7. Income 2.727(1.392)		.101	-.077	.128	-.330**	.091	.071	

table continues

Table 5.6 continued
Correlation matrix, means and standard deviations of selected independent variables and dependent variable total social work time costs (n = 77)

Variables Mean(SD)	1	2	3	4	5	6	7
				Variables			
8. Ethnicity .779(.417)	.157	.089	.168	-.050	-.110	-.122	.167
Total social work time costs 44.467(43.797)	.494***	.153	.104	.122	.336***	.139	-.125

Variables Mean(SD)	8
	Variables
Total social worker time costs 44.467(43.797)	.084

* p < .05, ** p < .01, *** p < .001

138

Table 5.8

Correlation matrix, means and standard deviations of selected independent variables and dependent variable total social work time costs: types of problems (n = 86)

Variables Mean(SD)				Variables			
	1	2	3	4	5	6	7
Problems							
1. Accommodation .302(1.107)							
2. Financial .686(1.647)	.053						
3. Adjust illness 1.291(1.827)	-.032	.082					
4. Family adjust .593(1.323)	-.036	.076	.312**				
5. Family relationship .337(1.080)	.474***	.378***	.301**	-.059			
6. Other relationship .302(1.041)	-.080	-.095	.089	-.080	.076		
7. Emotional 1.174(1.639)	-.029	.317***	.529***	.332***	.398***	.107	
8. Work or school .488(1.437)	.054	.399***	.156	-.006	.423***	-.068	.218*
9. Legal .267(1.067)	-.069	.396***	.153	-.005	.176	.096	.188*
10. Other .372(1.256)	.020	.000	.106	.135	-.016	-.087	.162
Total social work time costs 44.061(42.126)	-.139	.152	.115	.027	.129	-.047	.183*

table continues

139

Table 5.8 continued

Correlation matrix, means and standard deviations of selected independent variables and dependent variable total social work time costs: Types of problems (n = 86)

Variables Mean(SD)	Variables		
	8	9	10
9. Legal .277(1.062)	.489***		
10. Other .426(1.324)	-.102	.136	
Total social worker time costs 40.311(42.127)	.237*	.203*	-.098

* p < .05, ** p < .01, *** p < .001

Bibliography

Abramson, J. S. (1988), 'Participation of elderly patients in discharge planning: is self-determination a reality?', *Social Work*, Vol. 33, No. 5, pp. 443-448.

Abramson, J. S. (1990), 'Enhancing patient participation clinical strategies in the discharge planning process', *Social Work in Health Care*, Vol. 14, No. 4, pp. 53-71.

Abramson, J. S., Donnelly, J., King, M. A., and Mailick, M. D. (1993), 'Disagreements in discharge planning', *Health and Social Work*, Vol. 18, No. 1, pp. 57-64.

Afifi, A. A. and Clark, V. (1990), *Computer Aided Multivariate Analysis*, (2nd. ed.). New York: Chapman and Hall.

Ajzen, I. (1991), 'The theory of planned behavior', *Organizational Behavior and Human Decision Processes*, Vol. 50, pp. 179-211.

Berger, C.S., Cayner, J., Jensen, G., Mizrahi, T., Scesny, A., and Trachtenberg, J. (1996), 'The changing scene of social work in hospitals: A report of a national study by the Society for Social Work Administrators in Health Care and NASW', *Health and Social Work*, Vol. 21, No. 3, pp. 167-177.

Bergman, A., Wells, L., Bogo, M., Abbey, S., Chandler, V., Embelton, L., Guirgus, S., Huot, A., McNeil, T., Prentice, L., Stapelton, D., Shekter-Wolfson, L., and Urman, S. (1993), 'High-risk indicators for family involvement in social work in health care: a review of the literature', *Social Work*, Vol. 38, No. 3, pp. 281-288.

Berkman, B. (1996), 'The emerging health care world: Implications for social work practice and education', *Social Work*, Vol. 41, No. 5, pp. 541-551.

Bettman, J. R., Johnson, E. J., and Payne, J. W. (1990). 'A componential analysis of cognitive effort in choice', *Organizational Behavior and Human Decision Processes*, Vol. 45, pp. 111-139.

Blazyk, S. and Canavan, M. M. (1985), 'Therapeutic aspects of discharge planning', *Social Work*, Vol. 30, pp. 489-496.

Blumenfield, S. and Lowe, J. I. (1987), 'A template for analyzing ethical dilemmas in discharge planning', *Health and Social Work*, Vol. 12, No. 1, pp. 47-56.

Bray, N., Carter, C., Watt, J. M., and Shortell, S. (1994), 'An examination of winners and losers under Medicare's prospective payment system', *Health Care Management Review*, Vol. 19, No. 1, pp. 44-55.

Brown, J. S. T., and Furstenberg, A. (1992), 'Restoring control: empowering older patients and their families during health crisis', *Social Work in Health Care*, Vol. 17, No. 4, pp. 81-101.

Brown, R. S., Clement, D. G., Hill, J. W., Retchin, S. M., and Bergeron, J. W. (1993), 'Do health maintenance organizations work for Medicare?', *Health Care Financing Review*, Vol. 15, No. 1, pp. 7-23.

Campbell, D. T. and Stanley, J. C. (1963), *Experimental and Quasi-Experimental Designs for Research*, Boston, MA: Houghton Mifflin.

Carnevale, P. J., O'Connor, K. M., and McCusker, C. (1993), 'Time pressure in negotiation and mediation', In O. Svenson and A. J. Maule (Eds.), *Time Pressure and Stress in Human Judgment and Decision Making* (pp.117-127). New York: Plenum Press.

Carr, L. P. (1993), 'Unbundling the cost of hospitalization', *Management Accounting*, Vol. 75, No. 5, pp. 43-48.

Cleary, A. (1994, September 20). Boston, MA, 'The health care capital faces up to market-based reform', *Hospitals and Health Networks*, pp. 58-62.

Cleary, P. D., Edgman-Levitan, S., Roberts, M., Moloney, T. W., McMullen, W., Walker, J.D., and Delbanco, T. L. (1991), 'Patients evaluate their hospital care: a national survey', *Health Affairs*, Vol. 10, pp. 254-267.

Clemens, E. L. (1995), 'Multiple perceptions of discharge planning in one urban hospital',. *Health and Social Work*, Vol. 20, No. 4, pp. 254-261.

Concannon, K. W. (1995), 'Home and community care in Oregon', *Public Welfare*, Vol. 53, No. 2, pp. 10-16.

Cook, T. D. and Campbell, D. T. (1979), *Quasi-Experimentation. Design and Analysis Issues for Field Settings*. Boston, MA: Houghton Mifflin.

Cooper, R. (1990), 'Cost classification in unit-based and activity-based manufacturing cost systems', *Journal of Cost Management*, Vol. 4, No. 3, pp. 4-14.

Cooper, R. and Kaplan, R. S.(1991), *The Design of Cost Management Systems*. Englewood Cliffs, NJ: Prentice Hall.

Coulton, C. J. (1984), 'Confronting prospective payment: requirements for an information system', *Health and Social Work*, Vol. 9, No. 1, pp. 13-24.

Coulton, C. J. (1988), 'Evaluating screening and early intervention: a puzzle with many pieces', *Social Work in Health Care*, Vol. 13, No. 3, pp. 65-72.

Coulton, C .J. (1990), 'Research in patient and family decision making regarding life sustaining and long term care', *Social Work in Health Care*, Vol. 15, No. 1, pp. 63-78.

Coulton, C. J., Dunkle, R. E., Chow, J. C., Haug, M., and Vielhaber, D. P. (1988), 'Dimensions of post-hospital care decision-making: a factor analytic study', *The Gerontologist*, Vol. 28, No. 2, pp. 218-223.

Coulton, C. J., Dunkle, R. E., Haug, M., Chow, J., and Vielhaber, D. P. (1989), 'Locus of control and decisionmaking for posthospital care', *The Gerontologist*, Vol. 29, No. 5, pp. 627-632.

Coulton, C. J., Keller, S. M., and Boone, C. R. (1985), 'Predicting social worker's expenditure of time with hospital patients', *Health and Social Work*, Vol. 10, No. 1, pp. 35-44.

Cuzzi, L. F., Holden, G., Grob, G. G., and Blazer, C. (1993), 'Decision making in social work: a review', *Social Work in Health Care*, Vol. 18, No. 2, pp. 1-21.

Deakin E. B. and Maher, M. W. (1991), *Cost Accounting* (3rd. ed.). Homewood, IL: Irwin.

Demone, H. W. and Gibelman, M. (1989), *Services For Sale. Purchasing Health and Human Services*. New Brunswick, NJ: Rutgers University Press.

DeVellis, R. F. (1991), *Scale Development. Theory and Applications*. Newbury Park, CA: Sage.

Dobrof, J. (1991), 'DRG's and the social worker's role in discharge planning', *Social Work in Health Care*, Vol. 16, No. 2, pp. 37-54.

Doueck, H. J. and Bondanza, A. (1990), 'Training social work staff to evaluate practice: a pre/post/then comparison', *Administration in Social Work*, Vol. 14, No. 1, pp. 119-133.

Fein, E. and Staff, I. (1991), 'Measuring the use of time', *Administration in Social Work*, Vol. 15, No. 4, pp. 81-93.

Fischer, J. and Corcoran, K. (1994), *Measures For Clinical Practice* (2nd. ed.). Vol 1. New York: Free Press.

Foreman, P. (1964), Panic theory. In D. Schultz (ed.), *Panic Behavior*. New York: Random House.

Frankfort-Nachmias, C. F. and Nachmias, D. (1992), *Research Methods in the Social Sciences,* (4th. ed.), New York: St. Martins Press.

Garber, L., Brenner, S., and Litwin, D. (1986), 'A survey of patient and family satisfaction with social work services', *Social Work in Health Care*, Vol. 11, No. 3, pp. 13-23.

Grasso, A. J. and Epstein, I. (1993), 'Theoretical requirements for successful integration of information technology in human service agencies', *Child and Youth Services*, Vol. 16, pp. 17-32.

Greenley, J. R. and Schoenherr, R. A. (1981), 'Organization effects on client satisfaction with humaneness of service', *Journal of Health and Social Behavior*, Vol. 22, No. 1, pp. 2-18.

Haber-Scharf, M. (1985), 'Costing social work services in a hospital setting', *Social Work in Health Care*, Vol. 11, No. 1, pp. 113-129.

Hair, J. F., Anderson, R. E., Tatham, R. L., and Black, W. C. (1995), *Multivariate Data Analysis* (4th. ed.), Englewood Cliffs, NJ: Prentice Hall.

Hairston, C. F. (1985), 'Costing nonprofit services: developments, problems and issues', *Administration in Social Work*, Vol. 9, No. 1, pp. 47-55.

Hill, J. G. (1960), 'Cost analysis of social work service', in N. A. Polansky (ed.), *Social Work Research*, pp. 223-246, Chicago: University of Chicago Press.

Hogarth, R. (1987), *Judgment and Choice*. New York: Random House.

Homans, G. (1974), *Social Behavior*. New York: Harcourt, Brace, World.

Howard, G. S. (1980), 'Response-shift bias. A problem in evaluating interventions with pre/post self-reports', *Evaluation Review*, Vol. 4, No. 1, pp. 93-105.

Janis, I. (1982), *Groupthink: Psychological Studies of Policy Decisions and Fiascos* (2nd ed.), Boston, MA: Houghton Mifflin.

Janis, I., and Mann, L. (1977), *Decision-Making*, New York: Free Press.

Janis, I. L., and Mann, L. (1992), 'Cognitive complexity in international decision making', in P. Suedfeld and P. E. Tetlock, (Eds.), *Psychology and Social Policy*, pp.33-49, New York: Hemisphere Publishing.

Kadushin, G. and Kulys, R. (1993), 'Discharge planning revisited: what do social workers actually do in discharge planning?', *Social Work*, Vol 38, No 6, pp. 713-726.

Kasten, B. L. (1986), *The Physician's DRG Handbook*, St. Louis, MI: Mosby/Lexi-Comp.

Kayser, K., Hansen, P. and Groves, A. (1995), 'Evaluating social work practice in a medical setting: how do we meet the challenges of a rapidly changing system?', *Research on Social Work Practice*, Vol. 5, No. 4, pp. 485-500.

Keigher, S. M. (1993), 'Of dirty sheets and worse: administration costs and staffing matters', *Health and Social Work*, Vol. 18, No. 4, pp. 302-306.

Keller, S. M., Domanski, M. D., Macks, G., Manley, J. J., and Winder, D. E. L. (1993), *Productivity Measurement System for Administrators of Social Programs in Health Care*. Chicago: American Hospitals Association.

Kelly, H. H., Condny, J. C., Jr., Dahlke, A. E., and Hill, A. H. (1965), 'Collective behavior in a simulated panic situation', *Journal of Experimental Social Psychology*, Vol. 1, pp. 20-54.

Kendall, P. C. (ed.). (1991), *Child and Adolescent Therapy*. New York: Guildford Press.

King, M., Lapsley, I., Mitchell, F., and Moyes, J. (1994), *Activity Based Costing in Hospitals. A Case Study Investigation*. London: Chartered Institute of Management Accountants (CIMA).

Kirk, R. (1995), 'Managing the financial challenges of public-private collaboration', *Behavioral Healthcare Tomorrow*, Vol. 4, No. 2, pp. 31-34.

Klein, D., and Hill, R. (1979), 'Determinants of family problem solving effectiveness', in W. B. Burr, R. Hill, F. I. Nue, and I. L. Reiss, (eds.),

Contemporary Theories About The Family. Vol 1. pp. 493-538. New York: Free Press.

Knapp, M., Beecham, J., Anderson, J., Dayson, D., Leff, J. Margolius, O., O'Driscoll, C., and Wills, W. (1990), 'The TAPS project: 3: predicting the community costs of closing psychiatric hospitals', *British Journal of Psychiatry*, Vol. 157, pp. 661-670.

Lachman, R., Mistler-Lachman, J., and Butterfield, E. C. (1979), *Cognitive Psychology*, Hillsdale, NJ: Lawrence Erlbaum Associates.

Lawlor, E. F. and Raube, K. (1995), 'Social interventions and outcomes in medical effectiveness research', *Social Service Review*, Vol. 69, No. 3, pp. 383-404.

Lipshitz, R. (1993), 'Decision making as argument-driven action', in G. A. Klein, J. Oransanu, R. Calderwood, C. E. Zsambok (eds.). *Decision Making In Action:Models and Methods*, pp. 172-181. Norwood, NJ: Ablex Publishing.

Lockery, S. A., Dunkle, R. E., Kart, C. S., and Coulton, C. J. (1996), 'Factors contributing to the early rehospitalization of elderly people', *Health and Social Work*, Vol. 19, No. 3, pp. 182-191.

Manheim, L. M. and Feinglass, J. (1994), 'Hospital cost incentives in a fragmented health care system', *Health Care Management Review*, Vol. 19, No. 1, pp. 56-63.

March. J. G. and Simon, H. A. (1958), *Organizations*. New York: John Wiley and Sons.

Marcus, A. C. and Telesky, C. W. (1982), 'Non -participation in telephone follow-up interviews', *American Journal of Public Health*, Vol. 73, No. 1, pp. 72-77.

Marshall, G. M., Hays, R. D., and Mazel, R. (1996), 'Health status and satisfaction with health care: results from the medical outcomes study', *Journal of Consulting and Clinical Psychology*, Vol. 64, No. 2, pp. 380-390.

Morrisey, J. (1994), 'Higher costs in HMO-land', *Modern Healthcare*, Vol. 24, No. 26, pp. 102-110.

Moser, C. A. and Kalton, G. (1972), *Survey Methods in Social Investigation* (2nd. ed.). London: Heinemann.

National Association of Social Workers (1990), *Code of Ethics*. Silver Spring, MD: Author.

Neeson, H. R.(1996, January 15). *Professional Staff Update*, Boston, MA.

Nicholson, T., Belcastro, P. A., and Gold, R. S. (1985), 'Retrospective pretest-posttest analysis versus traditional pretest-posttest analysis', *Psychological Reports*, Vol. 57, No. 2, pp. 525-526.

Norusis, M. J. (1993), *SPSS for windows. Base System User's Guide, Release 6.0*. Chicago: SPSS Inc.

Nunnally, J. (1967), *Psychometric Theory*, New York: McGraw-Hill.

Oktay, J. S., Steinwachs, D. M., Mamon, J., Bone, L. R., and Fahey, M. (1992), 'Evaluating social work discharge planning services for elderly people: access, complexity and outcome', *Health and Social Work*, Vol. 17, No. 4, pp. 290-298.

Paese, P. W. and Sniezek, J. A. (1991), 'Influences on the appropriateness of confidence in judgment: practice, effort, information and decision making', *Organizational Behavior and Human Decision Processes*, Vol. 40, pp. 193-218.

Patti, R. (1987), 'Managing for service effectiveness in social welfare: toward a performance model', *Administration in Social Work*, Vol. 11, No. 3/4, pp. 7-21.

Pedhazur, E. J. and Pedhazur-Schmelkin, L. (1991), *Measurement, Design and Analysis: An Integrated Approach*, Hillsdale, NJ: Lawrence Erlbaum Associates.

Pilcher, D. M. (1990), *Data Analysis for the Helping Professions. A Practical Guide*, Newbury Park, CA: Sage.

Plous, S. (1993), *The Psychology of Judgment and Decision-Making*, Philadelphia, PA: Temple University Press.

Ponto, J. M. and Berg, W. (1992), 'Social work services in the emergency department: a cost-benefit analysis of an extended coverage program', *Health and Social Work*, Vol. 17, No. 1, pp. 66-73.

Poole, D. (1996), 'Keeping managed care in balance', *Health and Social Work*, Vol. 21, No. 3, pp. 163-166.

Proctor, E. K. and Morrow-Howell, N. (1990), 'Complications in discharge planning with Medicare patients', *Health and Social Work*, Vol. 15, No. 1, pp. 45-54.

Proctor, E. K., Morrow-Howell, N., Albaz, R., and Weir, C. (1992), 'Patient and family satisfaction with discharge plans', *Medical Care*, Vol. 30, No. 3, pp. 262 - 275.

Proctor, E. K., Morrow-Howell, N., and Lott, C. L. (1993), 'Classification and correlates of ethical dilemmas in hospital social work', *Social Work*, Vol. 38, No. 2, pp. 166 - 177.

Ramsey, R. H. (1994), 'Activity-based costing for hospitals', *Hospital and Health Services Administration*, Vol. 39, No. 3, pp. 385 - 396.

Reamer, F. G. (1985). 'Facing up to the challenge of DRG's', *Health and Social Work*, Vol. 10, No. 2, pp. 85-94.

Reid, W. J. (1987), 'Service effectiveness and the social agency', Administration', in *Social Work*, Vol. 11, No. 3/4, pp. 41-57.

Reinhardy, J. R. (1995), 'Relocation to a new environment: decisional control and the move to a nursing home', *Health and Social Work*, Vol. 20, No. 1, pp. 31-38.

Resnick, C. and Tighe, E.G. (1997), 'The role of multidisciplinary community clinics in managed care systems', *Social Work*, Vol. 42, No. 1, pp. 91-106.

Rosenberg, G. (1994), 'Social work, the family and the community', *Social Work in Health Care*, Vol. 20, No. 1, pp. 7-20.

Rosenfield, P. Kennedy, J. G., Giacolone, R. A. (1986), 'Decision making: a demonstration of the postdecision dissonance effect', *Journal of Social Psychology,* Vol. 126, No. 5, pp. 663-665.

Rosko, M. D. and Broyles, R. W. (1988), 'The financial impact of government on health services and administration: prospective payment systems and other regulatory programs', in J. Rabin and M. B. Steinhauer (ed.), *Handbook on Human Service Administration* pp. 215-241. New York: Marcel Dekker.

Rotter, J. B. (1966), 'Generalized expectancies for internal versus external control of reinforcement', (Whole Issue), *Psychological Monographs,* Vol. 80, No. 1.

Saffran, C. and Phillips, R. S. (1989), 'Interventions to prevent readmission', *Medical Care,* Vol. 27, No. 2, pp. 204-211.

Scott, L. (1994), 'Looking beyond cost', *Modern Healthcare,* Vol. 24, No. 9, pp. 36-39.

Semke, J., Stowell, M., and Durgin, J. (1993), 'Influences on social work time expenditure in a voluntary inpatient psychiatric unit', *Health and Social Work,* Vol. 18, No. 1, pp. 32-39.

Sheldon, B. (1986), 'Social work effectiveness experiments: review and implications', *British Journal of Social Work,* Vol. 16, No. 2, pp. 223-242.

Simon, E. P., Showers, N., Blumenfield, S., Holden, G., and Xiaochu Wu, (1995), 'Delivery of home care services after discharge: what really happens', *Health and Social Work,* 20, No. 1, pp. 5-14.

Smith, H. W. (1975), *Strategies of Social Research. The Methodological Imagination.* Englewood Cliffs, NJ: Prentice Hall.

Sniezek, J. A. and Buckley, T. (1993), 'Becoming more or less certain', in N. J. Castellan (ed.). *Individual and Group Decision Making: Current Issues,* pp. 87-108. Hillsdale, NJ: Lawrence Erlbaum Associates.

Spano, R. M. and Lund, S. H. (1986), 'Productivity and performance: keys to survival for a hospital-based social work department', *Social Work in Health Care,* Vol.11, No. 3, pp. 25-39.

Spano, R. M., Kiresuk, T. J., and Lund, S. H. (1986), 'An operational model to achieve accountability for social work in health care', *Social Work in Health Care,* Vol. 11, No. 3, pp. 123-141.

Svenson, O. and Edland, A. (1989), 'Changes of preferences under time pressure: choices and judgments', in H. Montgomery and O. Svenson (eds.). *Process and Structure in Human Decision Making,* pp. 225-236. New York: John Wiley and Sons.

Svenson, O. and Maule, A. J. (eds.) (1993), *Time Pressure and Stress in Human Judgment and Decision Making.* New York: Plenum Press.

Taira, F. and Taira, D, (1991), 'Patient 'dumping' of poor families', *Families in Society,* Vol. 72, No. 7, pp. 409-415.

Teisberg, E. O., Porter, M. E., and Brown, G. B. (1994), 'Making competition in health care work', *Harvard Business Review,* July-August, pp. 131-141.

Turban, E. (1990), *Decision Support and Expert Systems: Management Support Systems* (2nd. ed.), New York: Macmillan.

Vinter, R. D. and Kish, R. K. (1984), *Budgeting for Not For Profit Organizations*, New York: Free Press.

Volland, P. J. (1980), 'Costing for social work services', *Social Work in Health Care*, Vol. 6, No. 1, pp. 73-87.

Ware, J. E., Wright. W. R., Snyder, M. K., and Chu, G. C. (1975), 'Consumer perceptions of health care services: implications for academic medicine', *Journal of Medical Education*, Vol. 50, pp. 839-848.

Wicklund, R. A. (1974), *Freedom and Reactance*, Potomac, MD: Lawrence Erlbaum Associates.

Wolock, I., Schlesinger, E., Dinerman, M., and Seaton, R. (1987), 'The posthospital needs and care of patients: implications for discharge planning', *Social Work in Health Care*, Vol. 12, No. 4, pp. 61-76.

Zook, C. J., Savickis, S. F., and Moore, F. D. (1980), 'Repeated hospitalization for the same disease: a multiplier of National Health Costs', *Milbank Memorial Fund Quarterly*, Vol. 58, No. 3, pp. 454-471.